WHO AM I AND WHAT AM I DOING HERE?

Written by C.A. Smith

Copyright © 2020 by C.A. Smith
aka Christopher A. Smith

All rights reserved. No part of this book may be reproduced or used in any manner without the copyright owner's written permission except for the use of quotations in a book review. For more information, address: Chris@TheWellspringSenior.com

FIRST EDITION

Praise For
WHO AM I AND WHAT AM I DOING HERE?

"C.A. Smith has written a must-read for anyone aspiring to be a leader at the front lines in dementia care...Read this book - and learn from one of the best."

NATIONAL INSTITUTE FOR DEMENTIA EDUCATION
NIDE STANDARDS OF EXCELLENCE COUNCIL

"Dementia and other forms of neurodegenerative disorders are thieves. They steal the memory and mobility of our loved ones. Leading and working in places of care tests the limits of our compassion, as does any form of palliative care. It can provide us with moments of joy and love and in an instant bring down crushing chasms between us. In this marvelous and human book, C.A. Smith applies research-based principals of effective care and coaching to recreate a road map for us to make such settings feel like home."

RICHARD BOYATZIS, PHD
DISTINGUISHED UNIVERSITY PROFESSOR, CASE WESTERN RESERVE UNIVERSITY
CO-AUTHOR OF THE INTERNATIONAL BEST SELLER,
"PRIMAL LEADERSHIP" AND THE NEW "HELPING PEOPLE CHANGE"

"C.A. Smith has done a magnificent job of revealing the truth behind dementia patients and how they feel through their lens. Many times we treat dementia patients as their diagnosis, forgetting who they were and for many, who they still are, even if fragmented memories persist. As a senior industry leader myself, I am quite impressed at his ability to paint the picture very clearly so that the disease process is understood by layman which is so very needed in today's world of senior healthcare. I would highly recommend adding this literary work to your library, whether a paid caregiver or someone caring for a loved one at home. This book allows you, the reader, to step out of your own reality and for once, step into theirs."

SONJA GUNTER, LPN, AHS, ED
AUTHOR OF BOOK, "PROFESSIONAL TRAITS OF A HEALTHCARE LEADER"

"An inspiring book with a strong narrative – that does not just provide ideas but actionable strategies for anyone who works in senior care."

JOSHUA J. FREITAS, PH.D.(C), M.ED., BC-DED., ET AL
CHIEF RESEARCH OFFICER, CERTUS INSTITUTE CHIEF EDUCATION OFFICER, NIDE

"C.A. Smith easily outlines how to successfully implement a dementia care program, specifically the importance of support from the top of the company in order for a program to be successful—something we don't hear enough about! We specifically appreciate his push for online dementia training. If COVID has taught us one thing, it is to think outside the box, something C.A. Smith does in this book."

RACHAEL WONDERLIN, MS
OWNER, DEMENTIA BY DAY

"I loved the story; my interest was held initially, and I found it an easy read. I loved the family bond and how concerned they were for each other. I enjoyed the one point when the light bulb went off in my head, and I realized the title's double meaning. It kept my interest, was not too pretentious in explaining the business side, and understood the strategies C.A. Smith was trying to implement."

MARIA GRAZIANO
VETERINARIAN ASSISTANT AND MOM

"In this honest, inspiring, and informative book, author C.A. Smith encourages us to get to the heart of the matter to help redefine dementia care community culture together. The opening family narrative and the straightforward leadership strategy sections that follow share a human and compassionate message: to join, validate, and really listen to our care community at all levels, and to serve with passion and purpose, and without personal agenda. "

NATASHA GOLDSTEIN-LEVITAS, MA, BC-DMT
DANCE/MOVEMENT THERAPIST;
AGING AND DEMENTIA SUPPORT, COUNCIL MEMBER- NATIONAL INSTITUTE FOR DEMENTIA EDUCATION (NIDE) STANDARDS OF EXCELLENCE (SOE) COUNCIL

"An enjoyable book that was engaging and delightful and coupled with important information for those who need to care for those who can no longer care for themselves. You don't have to be in the senior care, dementia care, or leadership world to enjoy this book. It's wonderful."

CATHY BETHAM, RN
HOSPICE

C.A. SMITH　　　　　　　　　　　　　　　　　　　　WHO AM I AND WHAT AM I DOING HERE?

Dedication

I dedicate this book to every frontline professional caregiver who endures the frustration and anxiety of caring for those with dementia yet still find the compassion and love to return another day.
Matthew 25:40

To those with dementia - you are my friend.
1 Peter 5:7

To Maria, Cathy, and Jeanna - you are blessed and loved. Thank You for your investment in me. You are warmly appreciated.
Ephesians 1:16

And to Christopher and Angelina, who call me crazy, especially when I argue with myself.
Psalm 127:3

Table of Contents

PART ONE

Chapter One – The Discovery	1
Back To The Future	8
The Hurt	15
Perfect Timing	18
The Talk	22
Chapter Two – Who Am I?	25
Maxx and Duke	29
What Am I Doing Here?	33
Chapter Three – Duke's Wake Up Call; Time to Talk Some Business	37
Confronting Duke	37
Weekend With Maxx	40
Three Seconds to Vision	43
Follow Up Meeting	48
Chapter Four – The Maggie Plan	51
April 5th	51
Pet Peeves	56
Dementia Friendly Facility™	60
Introducing The Seven Strategies	65
The Funeral	72

PART TWO

Introduction 77

Chapter One 81
  Attitude And The Servant Leader 81

Chapter Two
  The Three Spheres of Focus 85
    Leadership - The First Sphere 86
    Marketing - The Second Sphere 89
    Training and Development - The Third Sphere 95

Chapter Three
  Seven Simple Strategies of Dementia Care Leadership ... 101
    Passion – The First Strategy 102
    Chameleon – The Second Strategy 107
    Vision – The Third Strategy 111
    Kaizen – The Fourth Strategy 116
    Effective – The Fifth Strategy 121
    Empowering - The Sixth Strategy 125
    Tribe, Teams, and Wolves – The Seventh Strategy ... 131

Appendix
  Recommended Leadership Books 135
  Don't Forget the Elephant 141
  Are you a leader? 142
  The WAG - Woodbridge Advisory Group 147
  Some of the Stories Behind the Story 149
  Final Thoughts 153

PART ONE

WHO AM I AND WHAT AM I DOING HERE?

Chapter One – The Discovery

A Splash of Pink Salt

It was the beginning of March 2020, and it seemed like the April showers started early. For Ginger, it was a bit colder than she likes. Her brothers, Maxx and Duke, would hear her frequently stating, "This Brooklyn, NY weather is not for me. My bones ache, especially when it's raining like this. Can't wait to go back to Florida."

"She should be here any second. She called about 30 minutes ago. I hope she gets here soon. I made some fresh coffee for her."

Ginger was talking with her brother Maxx on the phone, as she was looking out the window, "Oh, wait, she is pulling up right now. Maxx, let me go and hang up; I will see you later, OK?"

"Yes, sometime this afternoon. Do you need me there at a specific time?"

"No, anytime is good. I am not going anywhere. OK, bye."

Maxx hung up without saying goodbye. Ginger was so focused at the window so that she could open the door for Mishka, Maggie's nurse, not realizing that he hung up on her without saying goodbye.

"Wow, that's some storm!" Mishka exclaimed as she ran through the open doorway.

"I know! It's been windy and rainy for the past two days. Fortunately, it's supposed to stop tonight. But you know how it is, the weatherman is the only career that gets paid to be wrong all the time. How are you, Mishka?"

"Wet, but I am doing good. How about you, Ginger?"

"Well, you know, one day at a time."

"And how is our Maggie today? Have you noticed any changes in the past week since I was here last?"

"Well, a few changes, nothing that can't wait for a cup of coffee. Come into the kitchen. I have some freshly made croissants as well."

Ginger loved to entertain and always looked forward to the hospice and home care people to care for Maggie. It was the highlight of her day, even before her two brothers, Maxx and Duke, come over to visit.

"Besides, Lola, Maggie's aide, is still with Maggie freshening her up."

"Oh, that's good..." stated Mishka as she blew into the hot coffee. "I mean the coffee. It tastes perfect today."

"Well, I did something different today. I sprinkled a tiny dash of pink salt into the coffee maker. It neutralizes the bitterness and acidity and also enhances the flavor. I am testing how much - today was a sprinkle, tomorrow, maybe a dash," as she giggled.

"Not sure what the difference is between the two. But if you come by tomorrow, we'll find out together."

Mishka smiled as she enjoyed the coffee. "You know, I am going to try that myself. First a sprinkle, though."

"So, tell me what's going on. You said there had been some changes with Maggie. What kind of changes? And by the way, I love what you did to your hair. It's different."

"Well, thank you, you made my day!" exclaimed Ginger, with a spark in her voice. "Thank you! Maxx and Duke didn't notice, well they did, and in their defense, they came by on a small emergency with Maggie, and they were all focused on her."

"Emergency, what kind of emergency." Mishka focused her eyes on Ginger with intensity. The word 'emergency' in the hospice and home care business is not a 'good' word. Visions of police and ambulance and hospital visits started flashing in and out of Mishka's mind. Yet, with a cool calmness, before she took another sip of coffee, "You didn't tell me about any emergency?"

Ginger then realized that she was supposed to call Mishka about any and all emergencies without calling the police or ambulance. "It was small. Maggie rolled out of bed, and I couldn't get her back in. Maxx and Duke were here in a heartbeat. OK, well, 15 minutes, but they were here fast. They may not get along well, but they sure are here for Maggie when she needs them."

"When was this?", taking another sip, but a larger sip this time since the coffee was cooler.

"Oh, this was, let me see. Two days ago, just before the wind and rain."

Ginger was wondering if she was right. The days started to meld into one.

"Yeah, I am pretty sure it was two days ago. Don't worry; Maggie wasn't in any pain. Fortunately, we lowered the bed at night and have mats and cushions on the floor."

"Well, OK, so I will check her out. But I am sure one of the aides would have noticed something. Did you tell them that she fell?". Mishka was now concerned that one of the aides did not tell her that Maggie fell. They are supposed to report any changes or accidents of any kind, no matter how small.

"No, I did not tell them either. Probably because it was over the weekend, and I forgot. Sorry, Mishka - please forgive me."

"Oh! It's OK, Ginger, I understand. The days are combined, and it is hard to know what day it is and what happened on what day. Completely understandable. If it wasn't for the coffee," as she states with a smile and short giggle, "I think I would have a problem. Good thing for pink salt and coffee."

Ginger smiled with relief, "Don't forget the homemade croissants."

The Four Musketeers

Maggie, Ginger, Maxx, and Duke were all born and raised in Brooklyn, New York. In the Marine Park section. It was a mixture of Irish and Italians, most of which were Roman Catholics. Maggie was the oldest, born in 1950; Ginger was next in 1952, about 9 and 10 years later, came Maxx and Duke.

Their parents were typical of the time - diligent, hard-working people. Dad was a policeman, and mom was a stay-at-home housewife. Family life was good and pleasant with its routine ups and downs. Ginger, Maggie, Maxx, and Duke were affectionately called the 'four musketeers' by many parents in the neighborhood. Otherwise, nothing special here, except well ...

Duke has always been envious of Maxx, yet there was never a raging war between the two. Duke has high anxiety, almost with an attention deficit disorder, which was so common to diagnose in those days. Maxx used to say that A.D.D. means "always doing damage." Duke hated that phrase. Duke even hated when their father would say that the extra 'X' in Maxx's name meant 'extra' special. You see Maxx, had and still has a compassionate, even-tempered, and quiet-cool temperament. Whereas Duke, well, was almost A.D.D.

Maxx found school enjoyable and comfortable, always getting high grades. Maxx was good at starting and finishing high school and college projects. As a result, he started several businesses throughout the years, for example, in the 1970s, when the gas crisis and cars were lining up for hours at the gas pump. Maxx went out, bought bagels, spread cream cheese and butter on them, and sold them on the gas lines. He made a 'decent amount of money.' Duke helped out some too. But that's what Duke always did - he was always helping Maxx in some way or another.

Duke loved business too, but Maxx has an entrepreneurial leadership mindset, and Duke was more of a task-oriented person and enjoyed getting his hands dirty. He focuses on what he can do now and gets it done to mark it off his checklist. Unlike Duke, Maxx was patient. He carefully researched, planned, and then executed his plans. He believed that is the best way to eat an elephant, one bite at a time.

Maxx did have his failures in projects like the one where he tried to open up a computer school, invested thousands in a classroom and computers but did not do his homework with the marketing. The local high school started an adult education program that charged 1/3 of the price he was charging. They put Maxx out of business real fast. Interestingly, Maxx ended up managing and teaching the adult education program for that high school. Maxx thought it was a business failure with a silver lining. Duke thought it was a massive success for Maxx and was, well, a bit jealous.

Fast forward about 30 years, Maxx finished his doctorate in business administration and focused on human resources management. He headed a personnel department at Goldman Sachs in New York and taught as a Pace University professor.

Maxx wrote a book on people management that focused on the high stress and high anxiety world of finance. Maxx wrote the book to appeal to the executives in the finance field and was way "too detailed and intelligent for anyone else to read," as Duke would exclaim; "It's not for me, that's for sure."

Maxx lived quite well, staying in Brooklyn in the Mill Basin section, which was not too far from Marine Park, where Maggie lived, the home their parents raised them. They lived across the street from the elementary school where they all attended, P.S. 207. P.S. was the abbreviation for public school, but the kids said it meant "Pretty Stupid."

Duke never liked to visit Maxx, even though Maxx always invited Duke for dinner, especially during the holidays. Duke felt intimidated and insecure, so he stayed away. Duke wasn't the opposite of Maxx, and they did not hold animosity towards each other. They had their differences throughout the years, but there was never any big blowup or long years not talking. Not like the one that Ginger and Maggie had, the one they call 'the hurt' ... that went on for years.

It took Duke fourteen and a half years to finish his bachelor's degree at Brooklyn College. And that was after going to St. Francis college, first as a physical education major, then to Brooklyn College as a business major, then to Pace University as an accountant major to take the Certified Public Accountant exam. All the while working 10-12-hour days as a bookkeeper first at Prudential Bache Securities, then to JP Morgan and some other brokerage firms as a computer consultant. Duke loved that job because, as a consultant, he was his boss and made a "ton of money." Duke lived in Dyker Heights, Bay Ridge, Brooklyn, and is about 30 minutes from Maggie's apartment, depending on the traffic on the 'Belt Parkway.'

After Duke realized that accounting was not for him, "I couldn't sit at a desk all day and look at numbers. "I was going crazy," he frequently stated. He stopped school for a few years, "made some money and had some fun." As he was having fun, he got married and moved to Staten Island. He finished his bachelor's degree in business management and began working in the healthcare field with an up-and-coming home care organization. He first worked as a computer tech, but with his ability to work fast on task-oriented projects, he began to see how managing the aides and supporting staff would be something he would like. Over the years, he moved up the ladder, from manager to director to vice president and now C.E.O. and president. But Duke never viewed himself as a leader, especially when it came to running a company of 250 employees. Duke especially did not see himself as a success because he always compared himself to Maxx.

Ginger was the bright red head of the family. She was vibrant, active - not like Duke, busy but always looking for people to socialize with and carry on a conversation. She loved to talk. Yet, she never dominated the conversation, always eager to share and learn from others. She had natural strengths in being compassionate and empathetic. Both Maggie and Ginger were the same way in that respect. Ginger always referred to the two of them as "exact twins." Although there were some apparent differences between the two - especially when it came to 'the hurt.'

Ginger was a stay-at-home housewife to her husband. After 20 years of marriage, no children, he up and left and never came home. She suspects that he was cheating on her, but she did not know for sure. About five years after that, she received a request for divorce fully paid, and the house signed over to her with alimony.

She hinted that after five years, she was OK with it. She settled to the fact that she was never going to see her husband again. And then when the divorce paperwork came, well, it stirred up a whole bunch of 'whoop-ass' as she stated, and someone had to be the scapegoat. And that's when 'the hurt' started.

The divorce went through very fast, "I had nothing and nothing to protest. Gingers' ex was wrong. He knew it, and I guess that was his penance. I didn't have the energy to fight. I was in too much pain." So, Ginger moved things along as fast as she could so the pain would be over; so, she could forgive and move on.

After some time, Ginger moved to Florida, into a small, low maintenance home. She made some good money selling the house she was married in, 'the market was perfect for me,' she said as if the market had planned for her selling the home.

Ginger sold the home, took six months to travel, and then the market tanked. When she went to buy a smaller condominium, the prices were so reasonable that she didn't have to work another day in her life with the extra money she made on the house sale in Brooklyn and the alimony. Now she wasn't a millionaire and didn't have a whole lot of money saved, but Ginger lived a small and frugal life - so for Ginger, it was easy. As long as she had someone to talk with and share stories - she was happy.

Maggie, the oldest of the 'crew,' was in her early sixties when diagnosed with dementia. They think it may have been triggered by the anesthesia that she had in surgery after a car accident. In any case, they will never know.

Maggie was tall, about 5'10", thin and athletic. She enjoyed conversation just as Ginger did but was more interested in telling her story than she was in listening. Fortunately for Maggie, Ginger loved to listen. The two of them were almost inseparable until Ginger moved to Florida. Then Maggie, who never found the right husband, found herself alone.

Maggie worked in the healthcare field. First, as an I.C.U. Nurse, then as a home care nurse, and then as a hospice nurse. She said that being a hospice nurse "was a different world in healthcare, unlike any other nursing job." Not that she meant it was better or more demanding or more challenging - just different.

This 'difference' was always something that bothered her, and it wasn't until after she was diagnosed with dementia and planning the rest of the few years of her life with Maxx did she realize why it bothered her. So, she started making a journal about her days in the hospice world and how she felt about how things have been going on. About how 'business was done,' a term she learned from Maxx.

Maggie was always trying to express her feelings and had difficulty identifying what she was feeling and then putting them into words. At least not until she was diagnosed with dementia. Then she had a desire and a passion for writing everything down. Whether they made sense or not. And she knew that a lot of what she was going to write was not going to make sense. More importantly, she knew that she only had a short time left. So she wrote every day, and oddly the more she wrote, the more she felt, and the more she recalled. Especially when it came to the start of 'the hurt.'

Back To The Future

Ginger never really forgot about her husband leaving. This was way back somewhere in 2009. She may have forgiven him, but since there was no closure, no understanding why he left, she had trouble letting it go. Ginger had just come to settle into the notion that her husband was either missing, dead, or 'ran away with some floozy.' She didn't know which situation she preferred but was at a point in her life where she had to stop caring about him and move on. It was several years since the divorce was finalized. And the pain was pretty much gone, or at least she thought.

Ginger always dreamed of the day when her husband would come knocking on the door, she would cry, then 'smack him really, really hard in the face but not hard enough that it would leave a mark and then make love for the rest of her life with him.' At least that's what she told Maggie on more than several occasions.

But this time, it was different. Both Maggie and Ginger were at emotional times in their lives. Ginger had her ups and downs with her husband leaving, not knowing how to manage her finances, whether to sell the home or move back to Brooklyn and move in with Maggie. At the time, she worked as a cashier at the local Publix food market in Florida and barely making enough to get by.

Even though she was frugal and spared every penny, she still had trouble making ends meet. Every month, was a bounced check or insufficient funds fee. Not a whole lot but at least once a month, always borrowing from Peter to pay Paul. She joked, "Paul is looking for his money back." When she was speaking with Maxx in their weekly Sunday phone call together, she stated, "Maxx, this is the most stressful time in my life. I miss my husband's companionship, I am having trouble paying the bills, and I don't know what to do. Maxx, I am not asking for more money. Both you and Maggie have helped me with my finances already, which was more than I could ask. I am grateful that you listen."

The next day, they shut off her electricity.

Maggie had a different kind of stress. Her work as a hospice nurse was much more challenging than working as an I.C.U. nurse. "I just can't figure out what's wrong, but it bothers me, the interaction with the team. I mean, it doesn't feel like a team. Not like the teams I worked with at the hospitals. Even when I was a traveling nurse, it seemed like I was part of something bigger - I guess - oh, I don't know. I am having trouble putting my finger on it."

Ginger never knew how to respond but to listen when Maggie got this way. And Maggie didn't speak to Maxx and Duke. Duke didn't talk much to any of them. Not that he was mean or unsociable. That was just the way he was. Maggie justified it by saying that "Duke was not a talker. He was a doer - then she thought. He kinda likes to shoot first and ask questions later.'

Today was different; it was a Monday. Maggie was already trying to figure out how she could get Ginger out of this mess when she received the call from her director, early - real early at 7 a.m.

"Maggie, the aide for the patient in Sheepshead Bay, said you complained that your company is not doing a good job helping the family. And now the family is canceling the contract."

Maggie knows she did not say anything of the sort. There was some misunderstanding, but the director told her that she had to come to the office first.

She said, "It felt like she was marked as guilty and should come in for a hanging." Well, of course, Maggie was upset, distraught. She regularly reviewed her conversations with the family, the patient, and the aide. And since it was a full week ago, last Monday, she doesn't recall anything that would hint of that conversation.

Even before this event, Maggie was uncomfortable. She had to pull strings to get the social worker to help. She was always on the phone with the human resources department. She was in charge of making sure aides were scheduled with the patients, and the director was always complaining about some compliance issues. And not just to her, to everyone, and publicly through emails and weekly meetings. No-one was ever complimented or appreciated. "Every time I open an email or get a phone call, it's a complaint, problem, or issue."

Well, Maggie went into the office to find that Diane, the director of nursing, Dan, the director of the region, and Rachel, the representative for human resources, were present in the room. As soon as she walked in, she felt like her job was over.

The meeting began immediately with a barrage of questioning, mostly from Diane. It appeared Diane was not focused on a specific issue but seemed to be random. As if Diane was looking to blame Maggie for inconsistencies in the day-to-day activities at the office. Things she had no control over or responsibility for. Like scheduling the aides, coordinating with the social worker, and following up with phone calls over the weekends with the families. All of which were supposed to have been done by the director of nursing, who was on-call. It didn't make sense, and Maggie was confused.

"It seems that you are blaming me for the lack of follow-up that other staff members are responsible for. I was not on-call over the weekend in question, and I was not given access to the aides' schedules, and the social worker has not returned my calls - and Dan, I spoke with you about these very issues."

Maggie felt like a scapegoat and did not know how to react. She did think to get back to the issue, the call at seven this morning. "Dan, you called me at seven a.m. regarding a comment that the aide made. What did she say exactly?"

"Exactly? Wait, let me see."

As he was shuffling through some papers;

"Here it is, let me see, oh! She said to her boss..."

"Wait. What? Her boss? What do you mean?" Maggie said with a heightened and now more focused tone.

"Yes, her boss, the coordinator for the home care organization that hired her."

"So, you are not talking about our aide, Michelle?"

"No, I am not - it's an aide that the home care hired, and I think... wait, let me see, yup! It's an aide from another home care company - so it's a subcontracted aide." Just then, in a flash of a moment, Dan turned red as he realized what had happened and that he made a mistake. His face dropped.

Maggie then recalled the whole conversation. "I remember now. I talked to Michelle, our aide, about how the home-care company, the one the family pays privately and does not properly service the family. They don't show up on many occasions. I was asking Michele to keep an ear open because we need to make sure the patient is taken care of in the event they don't show up."

Relieved, Maggie relaxed with a big exhale.

Now Diane chimed in; that doesn't excuse the rest of the issues with your work. "And which issues are they specifically?" Maggie stated, frustrated and fired up.

"Never-mind. Dan, I think this meeting is over." Diane stated as she rose from her seat.

"Yes, I think so," He replied.

Maggie was in the room alone with Rachel, the human resources representative. Both of them looked at each other in amazement. As Rachel left the room, she stated, let me know if you need any help - and she was gone.

Maggie felt hurt, disrespected, and not cared for, and worse, unwanted. Even though she was with the company for five years, longer than anyone else, besides Dan, the director, she felt like she was trash. "How can a company that is supposed to serve and care for people be so insensitive to their employees? This place is like a revolving door. No one stays here - so what am I doing here?"

After that meeting, Maggie needed to relax for a few minutes, so she went to her car. Just as she was turning on some Christian music that relaxes her, Maxx called. "Hi, Maggie! How are you today?"

"Not too good. It's only 9:30 in the morning, I have yet to have my first cup of coffee, and I had a bad meeting with my boss - really bad. Are you interested in hearing about it?"

Even though Maxx and Maggie did not talk a lot, when they did, it always felt as if they talk every day. They get into the groove with each other fast. So, Maxx, who is always the good, compassionate listener, said, "Of course, I am all ears. Tell me what's going on."

So Maggie gave him the whole story from soup to nuts, almost verbatim. Especially the part where she feels like she does not matter.

Maxx said, "Sorry - that just plain sucks. It's unfair, and you should not be treated that way. You are a good person and do great work for people - you always have."

"Thanks, Maxx, I needed to hear that - Thank you! But I still don't understand, how can an organization, especially like hospice and home care, be so dis-compassionate?"

"Are you asking me for my opinion.?"

"Yes, Maxx, I am. You are my brother, with all the business sense. Tell me in plain English - what's wrong."

"Well, I don't know what is going on with your specific department or organization, but I have a good guess. Based on what I know about the senior health care business and what I see, it appears that they are compliance-focused and don't have a vision that will help employees like you, front line employees, realize a purpose and feel appreciated. Everyone needs to feel like they are part of a bigger picture, the vision - it's a basic human need. And I would bet 'dollars to donuts' that your director of nursing, your boss, Dan is it? And the human resources all feel that lack of purpose. Everyone exhibits it differently. It's bigger and much more involved yet, it's so simple - just love the people who work with you and for you. So that's my two cents."

"Hmmm," Maggie pondered and said, "so how do they stay in business. The turnover rate is high, and employee satisfaction is so low. And I know it's not just where I work. It's with other home care and hospice companies as well."

"That's easy. Because it's compliance-driven bottom-line focused. Productivity is based on the number of patients the organization brings on and keeps. Even though Medicaid or Medicare pays many and some insurances, those organizations don't look at employee satisfaction and turnover rate. The bottom line becomes a function of how well the required paperwork is maintained to get paid. It's an insurance and compliance-driven business, but I have a feeling it's not going to be that way for long."

"So, what about private pay families?"

Maxx said, "I would bet another dollar to donuts; hmmm, I could go for a jelly donut right now, wait, here's' a donut shop, I am going to pull right in and get one."

"Are you driving? You know you shouldn't be driving and talking on the phone."

"Yes, I am driving, but I have you connected to my Bluetooth."

"Wow, the connection is so clear, I couldn't tell."

"OK, sorry I digressed, back to donuts, I mean, private pay. The private pay people, I would guess, are referred by a doctor's office or hospital or something similar, so it is referral based. I would guess the education for those needing the care and those giving the care is lacking. I would think that the consumer needs more education in many different ways and continuously. And I would add, I bet most of the senior health care businesses that are not growing are the not well educated and not under-promising and over-delivering."

"You are right; I do not recall our company doing any kind of education in any manner to anyone, not even the staff. I just see them buying pizza and donuts for doctors' offices."

"OK," Maggie stated, "I have to say I am sorry, you called me for a reason, and I sabotaged the call. What's up?"

"It's fine, Maggie; I wanted to talk with you about Ginger. I am concerned about her situation. Ginger seems overly stressed and anxious."

"Yes, I agree, I spoke with her yesterday, and she does appear very anxious. I have been thinking about how to help her. But you know she brought a lot of this on to herself. She just sat and waited and waited and did nothing, hoping that that man would return. Always talking about her silly fantasy."

"Maggie, that's not fair. She's not you, and she handled it the best way she knew how. And I think it's sweet that she hopes for the best."

"Well, I still think she needs to get her head out of that dream and move on."

"I think she is moving on; she is just in a tough place right now. Hey, let me call you back later tonight. Is that all right with you?"

"Sure, Maxx - talk to 'ya later. Bye."

The Hurt

It's the end of the same day, about 4:30 p.m., and some of the other nurses are in the office writing some notes, updating charts, and making phone calls.

"Going to watch my daughter in a play tonight. Should be fun." Shouted one nurse.

"Really, what's the name of the play?" inquired the next nurse.

"Shrek - the musical. My daughter is playing Pinocchio. I saw it last night. She did great. She brought tears to my eyes. I am so proud of her."

Maggie added, "That's so nice. What a wonderful gift it is to have children. Well, for me, today has to be the worst day in a long time. I can't wait to get home, grab a glass of wine and sit in a hot tub and do nothing but relax and destress. Have a good night, ladies."

As she was heading home, Maggie tried to forget the morning events, but the more she tried to forget, the more heated up she felt.

"I am supposed to be calming down; what is this? Holy Spirit, please be with me and protect me from this anxiety."

She then put on her favorite Christian music, and her favorite song of all started to play, "What A Beautiful Name It Is."

As Maggie walked into her home, put her bag down on the side table, her keys on the key rack, and then removed her left shoe, the phone rang. It was Ginger. She thought, should I take the call or not?

"Oh, take the call," she thought to herself.

"Hi Ginger, how are you holding up today?"

"Not too good, can you talk?"

As she lifted her foot to take off the right shoe, she began to sit down to take off her sock. Her feet were pulsing as she rubbed them.

"Hold on a sec as I switch over to my headpiece. I just walked in the door."

"Oh, I can call you back if you want me to?"

"No, no, that's OK. I had a rough day and was going to sit in the tub and relax. So now is a good time. Talk to me."

Maggie then began to pour herself a glass of wine. She put the phone on mute, so Ginger can talk without being disturbed by the mild clashing of glasses and wine pouring. Just then, the wine bottle fell. It didn't break but spilled half the bottle onto the floor.

"Son of a bitch. I can't believe I did that. My only bottle of wine.! Son of a bitch!"

A moment later, "So am I going crazy or what?"

A pause...

"Maggie?"

Frustrated and angry, "Sorry, I forgot I put you on mute."

"Maggie, you sound upset. Did I say something wrong? Did I upset you?"

Ginger was cautious and sounded shaky in her voice. The last thing she wanted to do is upset Maggie. Maggie was all that Ginger had right now for comfort and support. They were not only sisters, but best friends, and Ginger needed Maggie.

"No, no, I am not upset." She said with a heightened tone. "Repeat what you said."

"I was telling you that I miss him and keep dreaming. I need him back."

Now Maggie was furious and blurted out;

"You know I am sick and tired of hearing you and your stupid dream, and your stupid husband."

She yelled louder, "He's not coming back. Get a grip; he's not coming back, so get your life in order."

Ginger was stunned at first, then began to feel darkness overcome her.

She hung up the phone.

Maggie realized what she said and felt horrible, but she wanted her wine, and it was all over the floor. "Damn it."

Something told her to call Ginger back right away.

Ring, ring, ring - no answer straight to voice mail.

"Ginger, I am sorry that was wrong. Call me back."

Maggie then went on to her nice hot bath, and the little bit of Cabernet left in her glass. She realized that she left her T.V. on in the living room, and in the background, she can hear, "Breaking News: This just in, Michael Jackson was found dead at the age of 50".

"Wow, I didn't know he was that young."

Perfect Timing

Ginger is sitting at home, going through her calendar, trying to plan the week. She always plans her week on Mondays, but today was different. She's running a bit late; she overslept or, more likely, didn't sleep at all.

"I must have eaten something that wasn't good for me," she whispered as she was checking off her to-do list.

"Taxes paid, check; grocery shopping, check; post office; Nah, it's almost 3 o'clock - I'll do that tomorrow."

Just then, a sweet melody came over her cell phone, a piano-playing 'somewhere over the rainbow.'

"Let's see who that could be...oh, it's Maxx."

"Hello, Maxx. How are you doing today? How's Brooklyn holding up without me there?"

"Fugetaboutit," he says in his natural Brooklyn tone. "I am doing good. A lot of rain, though. Everything is wet - this April showers, ya' know. Hey, just wondering if you heard the news. There was a bombing at the Boston Marathon a few minutes ago."

"No, I haven't. Was anyone hurt?"

"Not sure; it's still new. Hey, I haven't brought this up in a while, well. Are you going to let Maggie back into your life? It's been four years. I know she wants to talk and get back to the way things were between the two of you."

"Well, I don't think things will be the same, but I was going to call her today. I just wrote it down on my calendar. I agree; I think it's time. Four years is a long time, and I think I may have punished myself more than I thought I was punishing her."

"That's good to hear. If you want to talk, I will be here for you - just like always. And hey! Come visit... I still have room for you here. It's been a long time."

"OK, Maxx, I think that might be a good idea. One step at a time. Goodbye."

Ginger has been thinking long and hard for weeks now and realized that today is the day. "Hmmm, maybe that's why I didn't sleep."

Ginger waited until 6 p.m. when she knew that Maggie would be home from work, or at least it would be a good chance that she would be home.

"OK, here we go, 6 0 9 4 5 1; wait, that's not it, oh! I forgot about it. I will never get used to these cell phone things. I should have never removed that phone line last month.

OK, let me see, oh, there she is."

The phone was ringing. Ginger was anxious but less anxious than she thought she would be. She wanted this to be over too and get back to the way things were. As the phone rang, she wondered, "Can things be back the way they were?"

"Ginger?" Maggie quietly said with a pause..., "hello?"

"Hi, Maggie, it's Ginger."

"I know, I know!" muddled Maggie with a frog in her throat.

"I miss you, Maggie, I miss you so much."

"I miss you too, Ginger," tears started slowly flowing as Ginger had trouble getting the words out.

"I am so sorry, so sorry... please forgive me. I love you so much."

"I do forgive you, and I love you too, Maggie. Will you..."

It was only a few seconds pause, but it seemed like hours.

"Will you forgive me?"

"Stop, there is nothing to forgive. I love you."

"I love you too," said a relaxed Ginger. "How are you? How is Brooklyn and work, and I miss you, Maggie!"

Maggie replied with a tear flowing down her cheeks, "Brooklyn is wonderful. But it's raining for two days, but it's the sunshine, and I miss you so much. And work, well, I had to find another company to work for, same business, hospice, kind of except they do home-care as well. Tonight, I am on-call, which means I have to keep the phone with me all night into tomorrow at 5 a.m."

"I know it's raining a lot. I was on the phone with Maxx earlier today. He is tired of it too."

Maggie and Ginger talked on the phone for hours, as if they had never stopped and finished just before midnight.

"Can I call you later this week, Maggie? Maybe Saturday? I am sure we missed a few things so that we can do more catching up."

"That sounds great; let's do it. I plan to be home all day Saturday and Sunday. I am looking forward to it. Oh! Ginger, I love you! And miss you so much."

At that very moment, Maggie's work phone rang, "Well, look at that. Perfect timing, it's the on-call triage nurse. She only calls when I have to go out to visit a patient. I have to get this. Good night Ginger, love you."

"Good night Maggie, I love you too."

As soon as she got off the phone, Ginger thought she would take Maxx up on his offer. She was going to fly in from Florida and surprise him this coming Saturday.

"I am going to book a flight, first thing in the morning. Right now, it's almost midnight, and I have a list of things to do tomorrow." Ginger thought.

Ginger was dreaming of the song, "Somewhere Over The Rainbow," then she woke up. Her phone was ringing that same tune.

It was Maggie, at 3:27 in the morning?

"Maggie? Are you OK?"

"Hello, ma'am. This is Officer Reilly, with the New York Police. You are listed on Maggie's phone as the I.C.E. person. Is that true?"

"What, the officer who? What does I.C.E. mean?"

"Sorry ma'am, Officer Reilly. And I.C.E. means, 'In Case of Emergency.' You are on Maggie's phone as..."

"Emergency, what do you mean?"

"There has been an accident, a car accident. Maggie lost control of her car, and well, she is in the hospital. Can you get to Coney Island Hospital? She will need you. I am told she will be going into surgery."

"Oh, my, no, I am in Florida. But I will be up right away. I will call my brother, Maxx. He lives close by and will get there right away."

Ginger hangs up without saying 'goodbye.'

"Where is his number? Oh, "stop shaking," as she says, "now I'm scared." Wait, he just called; there it is in the recent calls list."

Ringing... ringing...

"Come-on, Maxx, pick up. Oh, not voice mail."

"Let me try again..."

"Oh, he's calling back... Maxx, Maggie was in a horrible accident, and she is at the Coney Island Hospital. Can you get there right away?"

"Ginger, I am already on the way; I got a call too. Stay by the phone, and I will call you right back."

The Talk

"Ginger, I think you are right; we should talk to her and get her tested. It's been almost 18 months since her accident. She has been slowly declining. I will talk to her."

"OK, Maxx. Let's do this together this Sunday. I will fly up, wait, I think I will drive up and stay a few weeks, maybe a month. What do you think?"

"Ginger, I think that is going to be a great idea. Maggie is going to need you, now more than ever. We can figure things out during that time."

Sunday

"That was a great meal," said Duke after a well-deserved burp. "Excuse me."

"Yeah, I haven't had lamb in a long time. So happy that you came up and cooked for us, Ginger. Remember the days when we used to go around the corner to the butcher, and put in a special order for a leg of lamb." Maxx recalled.

"That's when you used to call me 'the Duke'ster.' Yeah, we were just kids. Memories."

"I'm full, but if you have dessert, I think I can find room. Wait for it, wait for it." Burp... 'excuse me. I have room now."

"Duke, you're such a kid sometimes; if someone didn't know you ran a 250-person healthcare company, they would never find out from this wonderful dialog."

"Maxx, I think I feel like a kid. My brothers and sisters are all together, we have lamb and wait, I think I see, cannolis, sfogliatelle, and is it... yes, zeppole. Now, I am in heaven."

"Ginger, is there a limit on the zep's, and..., on the cannolis, and sfogliatelle, too?"

"Yes, you know the rules. One each, and after everyone has had one, and you want another one, you have to ask everyone first."

"Ginger?"

"Yes, Duke?"

"Did you get the authority from the Italian consulate to make zeppole's other than St. Joseph's day, March 19? Ya' know those are the rules?"

"Stop busting my chops and eat."

"Love you, Ginger."

"Just eat."

Ginger then yelled out to Maggie, who just finished washing the dishes, "Maggie, come out here. Later, we'll finish cleaning up together. Besides, God made dishwashers so we can talk more after dinner. Come enjoy it with us."

"Well, OK, OK, mommy. I am almost done with the dishes! I'm coming." Maggie giggled on the way back to the table.

"Sometimes, you sound just like a mom... but I love it."

"Maggie. Duke, Maxx, and I wanted to talk with you about something."

"OK, I am listening. I hope I didn't do anything wrong. Besides. I have to get started doing the dishes; they are piling up."

Duke, Maxx, and Ginger looked at each other. Maxx lost his appetite, Ginger didn't have one, and Duke, well, he was on his third zeppole.

"Duke, wipe the sugar powder off your mustache.", Ginger commanded.

"Oops."

"Maxx, would you like to start?"

"Sure, Ginger, I will. Maggie, we wanted to talk to you about going back to visit a doctor. A special doctor. It seems that you have been getting a little forgetful, and we want to make sure that there is nothing wrong. Just a routine checkup."

"I know, I know. I have been thinking about the same thing. Even at work, it seems that I have been making a lot of mistakes in the past month. I was written up twice. One more, and I am fired."

"Maggie, I didn't know that," whispered Ginger, as if it was a secret.

"Sorry, I didn't tell you, Ginger. I was ashamed and embarrassed. After the accident and the surgery, I think that I might be getting Alzheimer's or dementia or something. Something isn't right."

"Maggie, why didn't you talk to us. We are all here for you. All of us - even Duke." Maxx was trying to lighten the mood with no success.

Duke and Maggie both worked in the healthcare field. Duke's business is in hospice, home care, and close ties with a local assisted living center. Maggie worked as a hospice and home-care nurse, and Maxx, well, he knew enough from the conversations over the past two or more decades, and two of his older friends were diagnosed with dementia. One died about six months ago. Dementia was close to home, and everyone knew the outcome.

"Maggie, we love you, and we would like you to talk to us about what is going on. Please tell us everything."

"I agree, Ginger is right. We will be here for you, every step of the way."

"Thanks, Maxx."

"Maggie, every resource that I have will be at your disposal. You will never suffer from want or need."

"You see, even Duke can break away from a zeppole to help. If he can do that, he can do anything."

They all giggled and smiled warmly at Maggie.

Chapter Two – Who Am I?

Who Am I?

"What are you doing? Maxx."

"Hi!, Ginger. I was just looking through Maggie's journal that she started writing after she was diagnosed. Do you realize it's been almost two years since she was diagnosed? Anyhow, there's a lot of insight here. Since she was in the healthcare field, she was sensitive to the way people took care of her. I thought this would note about regrets, loves, passions, but it's not. She wasn't happy with the way things were in the business that she worked. And we are talking about Duke's field. I mean not his particular business but the industry. I want to look more into this and talk with Duke."

"OK, Maxx, she hasn't left us yet - so can you put your leadership and business hat someplace else and save this for later. I need help with moving Maggie into the living room. It's almost time for our New Year's Eve dinner. Besides, Maggie said you could read that after she's gone."

"Sorry, it was not intentional. I just got pulled into it. I will save it for later."

Maxx quietly entered Maggie's bedroom. Maggie was in the fetal position, looking up and smiling from the corner of her mouth. She was just 'freshened up' by our live-in aide, Lola. Lola was an employee of Duke's home care company. 'The best in the company,' said Duke as she came to interview her first time.

She was short, about 5 foot 3 inches, stocky, with a pleasant smile - a perpetual smile, all the time. Lola had a strong personality too. She took full ownership and control of Maggie's care. She once stated in her Jamaican tongue, 'Mi nuh kin teet' or 'I don't play around' when talking about loving her job and taking it seriously.

Lola once stated, "I get the privilege and the honor of using the gifts that God gave me to care for other people, like Maggie and her family. And the best part is, I get rewarded every day with love. It's the best job in the world, and God gave it to me."

Ginger enjoys Lola's company and companionship, especially when Ginger compliments her about ten times a day, and Lola replies in her Jamaican accent,

"Yuh suh sweet, tank yuh!"

"Maggie, it's time to go in the living room.", as Ginger lightly removed the sheets from Maggie.

"Who am I?" Maggie asked with a whisper.

"What?" responded a stunned Ginger.

"Why you're Maggie, my sister. And Maxx is your brother. You're his sister too."

"Who am I?" she asked again, but this time a bit louder and with more of a question behind the tone.

"Oh, Maggie...!" sighed Ginger.

"Come on, Maxx, ready?"

"Yup."

"OK, on three, one, two, three..."

"Upsee-daisy. There we go, Maggie. Now we can wheel you into the living room to hang out with us. I called the first New Year's kiss."

"Who am I?" Maggie shouted after arriving in the living room.

"You are Maggie!" offered Maxx.

"Whose Maggie? Maggie?"

Staring Into Space

"Well, that's new, Maxx. Hasn't she asked that question before? She's started to decline a lot in the past two or three weeks. At least with her personality. It's like she's losing hope or purpose in her life and giving up. I know that's not what is happening. It's a product of dementia, but it's so hard for me to understand some days. Some days are harder than others, and hearing her say that, well, it hurts. I hurt for her - yet she doesn't seem to be hurt. Do you know what I mean?"

"I think I do, Ginger, I think I do. I guess we are trying to rationalize a process that is not rational. It doesn't make sense. I know it's been a couple of weeks that I have visited. I am sorry."

"No, it's OK, you have been away on business. So, how is that working for you?"

"Well, I love the business of consulting. It was a good career move, and three years into it, I have set up a nice groove of making my schedule. And I can be picky about the companies that I work with, and it looks like I am naturally gravitating to senior healthcare, and it looks like the business of dementia care is a passion. It is an entirely different field and much more challenging. And I think that's why I like it. Helping leaders, at all levels, take a higher place and focus on relationships and people. I do enjoy it. When those light bulbs come on, and the directors and managers turn into leaders - it's a big payoff for me.

But you don't want to hear about the business. I am back and here to be of whatever support I can.

Oh, I received a call from a large dementia care organization in Florida, something called 'Sunshine Dementia,' I think. They wanted to hire me to help transform the company. Since that's your home state, I thought you would be interested."

"Never heard of them, what part of Florida."

"Oh, I don't know the details yet. I received an email from another consultant this morning. She seems to do the same kind of leadership work as I but in the construction business. I will find out more next week.

So, tell me about the last two weeks. What's going on with Maggie?"

"Well, it was about two weeks ago, no maybe three, when I started noticing her stare into space. Not for a few minutes but for an hour or so at a time. Well, you just saw her when we went in to pick her up. She was staring into nowhere, and now, when she comes out of it, it takes her more time to look at me."

"Well, that's discouraging and upsetting too, I am sure."

"It hurts, Maxx. I don't think she knows me anymore. It's like she's letting me go or, well, like she's all packed and leaving forever. I am afraid of losing my best friend."

Ginger was having a rough day; tears and emotions were on and off. Fortunately, Maxx was able to offer her a compassionate ear and companionship. Except for Lola, Maxx has been the only one who visits and stays.

"Duke comes by, once or twice a week, but he only stays for 30 or 40 minutes. And since Maggie sleeps so much - oh!"

Ginger pauses for a moment...

"I forgot to tell you that as well."

"Tell me what?"

"That she is sleeping a whole lot more. So, Duke doesn't stay much because Maggie is sleeping and only wakes up for a few minutes."

"Sorry, Ginger, would you like me to speak with Duke? He needs to realize that he should be visiting you more often. He just needs a good nudge in the right direction. He is so task-oriented that he needs to put visiting you on his list. It's just the way he operates."

"No, I don't want to embarrass him. Don't need another 'hurt' happening, that's for sure."

"OK, I will try to slip it gently into a conversation about it. How about this, why don't I try to get Duke to come with me. I will make a special trip. He needs to know. We will do it in a gentle way that's comfortable for both of you."

"Well, OK, I trust you will be gentle, for all of us."

"So, what else has been going on? Is Lola, well, still Lola?"

Maxx and Duke

A few days later, Maxx invited Duke to lunch at 'The Grand Marnier restaurant' in downtown Brooklyn. At night, it's a romantic place to bring your loved one, but during the day, it's pure business with the dining room full of suits.

It was Maxx's favorite French restaurant with 'butter galore.'

"This is a nice treat, Maxx."

Just then, they were pleasantly interrupted by the waiter,

"Pardon, monsieur. May I get you something from the bar?"

"Duke?"

"Nothing for me. Can I get a bottle of San Pelligrino, please?"

"And I will have a bottle as well, S'il Vous plaît," added Maxx with his try at the French language.

"So how is Maggie? I feel bad that she has declined so much recently. She sleeps all the time."

"Yeah, you know how it is. It's part of the process."

"Unfortunately, I do know, but not as well as I should."

"What do you mean, Duke?"

"Well, can we talk about my stuff later? Let's talk about Maggie. I miss her."

"I do too. Can we talk about Ginger, first?"

"What? What's wrong with Ginger?"

"Nothing is wrong with Ginger. I just think she is lonely, and she misses Maggie too, even though she cares for her all day, every day.

I was there the other day, and she seemed to need companionship and someone to talk with besides Lola. And then there's this new thing..."

Duke put his glass down and focused intently... "Yeah, I am listening."

"Maggie doesn't know who she is anymore. She keeps asking, 'Who am I?' It's almost all the time now. Seems like she lost her identity, her purpose, or hope."

"That's heartbreaking," Duke sighed and paused for a while, "Makes us realize how delicate life is."

"Duke, what are you doing tonight?"

"No plans, well a conference call at six but after that I am free. What are you thinking?"

"Invest a few hours with Ginger, Maggie, and myself. I will pick you up, let's say 6:45, and if you are still on the call, I can wait."

Maxx didn't give Duke any chance of saying no or come up with an excuse.

"Good plan; I like being chauffeured by you. It feels special. You're on!"

"You like those French words."

"Huh?"

"Chauffered..."

"Cute... real funny. Hey, how is the consulting work going? Still doing leadership stuff with those brokerage firms, no wait, you switched, didn't you?"

"Yeah, it's kinda taking a natural turn for me into the senior and dementia healthcare field. I guess because of Maggie's' condition, and I have been researching dementia care. What's good about leadership development is that it's more about people instead of a particular business. I mean, there is a learning curve when understanding the nuances of a specific industry..."

"There goes the French.", Duke interrupted.

"Huh?"

"Nuances, that's French. Isn't it?"

"Yes, Duke, you are right."

"So, where was I, oh, nuances. If I were doing management consulting, for me, there would be more of a need to focus on the industry specifics, but with leadership consulting, well, there is more of a... 'Je ne sais quoi'..."

"Oh, come on. You said that on purpose."

"Yeah, but not sure if I used it correctly. I had too..."

"What I meant was there is more flexibility because people are people, and I enjoy helping leaders get out from behind their desks and tasks and focus on the people. I like to think I specialize in servant leadership, and I think it's going to be in the dementia care field."

"That's what I need to do, get out from behind my desk. I need that management to leadership mentality. I always feel stuck and behind the eight ball. It's frustrating. I had turned into the micro-manager I always hated when I was working up the ladder. It's such an unproductive place to be."

"Well, if you want help, let me know, we can talk. Initially, it would require more talk. Duke, I am very picky about my clients and who I serve. If the individual is not committed to change, then I don't take them. I need that 110% commitment to change. Many managers and directors say they want it but are not in the place to change."

"Well, let me think about it, Maxx."

"There you go. That statement tells me where you are. You are not ready yet. That's fine, and that doesn't mean you won't be. This stuff takes time. Let's keep talking about it."

"I may be taking on a big job in Florida; it's a healthcare company that specializes in home-care and hospice. They specialize in dementia care. Well, I misspoke, not yet; they want to transform their company into a dementia centered company - they are looking at the projections for the growing demand in dementia care over the next 10-20 years, and they want to be ready. It takes time, and they want to be in front of it. I get the impression they have some challenges in leadership that they need to overcome. I am going down next week. These projects take time. If I take it on, it's going to last at least a year, if not two. Let's see what happens. The whole world could change between now and well, whenever you are ready."

"Sounds interesting, and I am intrigued. I would like to hear more as time moves on. How is that chicken cutlet? Looks good."

"It is delicious. Buttery soft, and the garlic mashed potatoes are good too. Hey, you getting dessert?"

"No, I have to get going as soon as we finish. I have a meeting with the compliance department - the bane of my existence. Hey Maxx, if you had one book, one book only to recommend, what would that be."

"Oh, for you and what we just talked about, "Good to Great." Read it, then listen to it, then read it, then listen to it again. Then come back to me, and we can talk. Give yourself time and let it absorb. Once you find your seat on the bus, we can talk."

"Huh, bus? I'm not getting on a bus."

"Just read it. If you want, I will give you my copy."

"No thanks, Maxx. Barnes and Noble is on the way home; I will get it there. "Good to Great"?"

"Yes, it has a red cover. James Collins is the author. You can't miss it."

What Am I Doing Here?

Maggie was awake this morning but tired. Chloe, another aide - the fourth this year, had just finished cleaning up Maggie and changing the sheets when Mishka, the case manager, and nurse knocked on the door.

"Good Morning, Mishka. How are you today?" said a tired Ginger.

"Trying to get through this weather. You are from Florida, aren't you? Hurricane Michael did some serious damage there yesterday. Any relations or people you know? Is everyone all right?"

"Thanks for asking. No, I have no relations down there. Everyone is here in Brooklyn. I still have a place down there but haven't been there in two years. I have someone looking after it, and he says there was no damage. I was worried, though. I think I will sell it, but maybe later - oh! I don't know."

"So, how is Maggie today?"

"The past week, she has been doing well. She seems more alert too. Sleeping about the same, maybe 15 - 18 hours a day. We haven't seen the decline in her that we had seen earlier in the year. We had a few scares when we thought we were going to lose her."

"Yes, Ginger, I remember. How is she eating?"

"She is doing good. Still soft foods, thickened liquids, she loves her apple sauce. Oh, and of course, ice cream too. You know what's interesting, she stopped asking, "Who am I?". The last time she said it was maybe two or three weeks ago. I just realized that - hmmm."

"Does she talk at all?"

"Oh yeah, earlier in the day, she is more understandable, but later in the day, if she talks, it's word salad with only a few words that are clear, if that many.

Yesterday, she was talking about when we went to the beach when we were young. 'Riis Park,' she kept saying, 'Riis park.'"

"Hi, Chloe," said Mishka as she walked into Maggie's bedroom. "How is our friend today."

"She is doing well. Very responsive and cooperative today. She was a joy to care for. She said she wants to go to the beach and play in the sand."

After about 30 minutes...

"Well, Ginger, things are going well. All vitals are good - nothing to report. But I do have to talk with you. Can we sit?"

"Sure, would you like a cup of coffee and danish," Ginger said as she was already pouring a cup.

"Well, since you already poured it - thank you."

"Ginger, I love Maggie, and I have grown to love you as well. Unfortunately, I am moving on and going to California to be with my family."

"Oh! Mishka, that is so nice of you. I am so happy for you. Good for you! Let me hug you!"

"Thank you so much. Now I don't know what is happening with a new nurse. I gave my notice three weeks ago, and they still have not made any plans. So, I would guess one of the nurses who works with my team would be checking in until they get a new nurse."

"Wow, that means more change. You know Maggie does not do well with change."

"I know, and I am so sorry. I tried to work with management, but our regional director was replaced twice in the past year, and I was having trouble getting them to listen. It seems that they don't hire people who care about the front lines. These past two directors, I only saw once each."

"Mishka, I have noticed a change in the company. The aides changed five or six times, and they never called me to tell me. Chloe is great, perfect, but I am afraid that they are going to take her away. Maggie needs stability in her relationships."

Mishka gently offered, "Ginger, if I may be so bold, I know Maggie's brother, Duke, is the C.E.O. May I suggest you talk with him. I have a strong feeling he is not aware - or maybe no-one is talking with him. And in his defense, the office seems to be focused on compliance this year. So, I would guess he is overwhelmed. I am not sure. Maybe a gentle conversation, well, he might listen to you, both of you."

"OK, I, I mean, we, both Maggie and I, will talk to Duke. But I am so happy for you, California. Which part?"

After an hour of pleasant conversation, Mishka and Ginger go in to see Maggie. Maggie was sitting up, in her recliner, awake but staring into space.

"Chloe, I didn't know you wanted to put her in the recliner. I would have been more than happy to help.", mentioned Mishka in a soft but authoritative tone.

"Maggie, Mishka is coming back to say hi. She came to say, oops, I almost did say it..."

"Said what, Ginger," responded Mishka in a concerned voice.

"I understand that if you say 'good-bye' to someone with dementia, it leaves a space or a lost connection. It might cause anxiety or confusion. So if we say, 'see you in a little bit,' or 'see you soon,' there is still a connection. That's what I learned, but I am not sure if that is the case with Maggie - in her present condition."

Mishka nodded her head, "Oh, I did not..."

"What am I doing here?" yelled Maggie. "What am I doing here?" she yelled as clear as if she didn't have one bit of dementia.

Ginger, Mishka, and Chloe each looked at each other in amazement. What did this mean? They silently asked each other.

Later that early evening, about 6 p.m...

"I don't understand. Then Maggie started to cry and repeat it. Several times today. Maxx, I don't know what this means."

"I don't know either - beats me. Maybe Maggie has a memory that kicked in or something. Well, let me see her. Is she sleeping?"

"Probably, I will go with you. Hey, is Duke coming?"

"Yes, he said he would be here in a little while."

Maggie was sound asleep, resting like a little child.

"She is so precious, Maxx. So precious."

Maxx put his arms around Ginger as Chloe softly left the room so Maxx and Ginger could be alone with their sister.

Knock knock... "Someone is at the door. I will get that," said Chloe.

"Hey, guys!" shouted Duke, "How is our bucket of sunshine today?"

"Hi Duke, she is most certainly different, but still our bucket of sunshine.", responded Ginger.

"What do you mean different?" exclaimed Duke.

"Let's sit down together, later," mentioned Maxx. "I have a business to talk about with Duke, but first Maggie."

"I knew it was going to be a long night, so I bought some pastries and cookies," said Duke.

"Thanks, Duke," Ginger exclaimed as she placed the desserts on a dish.

"So what's happening, guys?" notes Duke to move things along.

For over two hours, the three siblings talked about growing up and good times together. They talked about Riis Park, probably because Maggie brought it up, and Buddies Playground on Flatbush, Lenny and John's Pizza, the Copper Penny Restaurant, playing stickball and listening to the Steve Miller Band while playing pinball machines.

They also talked about the inevitable and how Maggie would soon graduate. The funeral and memorial services and how it was all prepared by Maggie, a few months after being diagnosed.

Chapter Three – Duke's Wake Up Call; Time to Talk Some Business

Confronting Duke

"Ginger, I would like to talk business with Duke. Is that OK?"

"Is it about what we talked about earlier, the changes?"

"Well, to start, yes."

"OK. I will go upstairs and get ready for bed. It's 10 o'clock. Almost past my bedtime."

"Thanks, Ginger.", Maxx sighed.

Both Duke and Maxx sit down in the living room.

"Duke, at the beginning of the year, we had lunch. Remember at "The Grand Marnier" restaurant. You asked me about a book, "Good to Great."

"Yes, I remember. Great book - pun intended."

"Well, along those lines, I wanted to talk with you about Maggie. Not sure if you know, but Maggie, well, dementia patients, in general, do not take well to changes. Especially in the care staff."

"Yes, I do know that. What does that have to do with Maggie? Is everything all right?".

"Well, no. Over the past six months or so, there have been a half dozen changes in the home care staff and the hospice aides. Now we understand there have been two changes in the past 12 months in the regional director. The case manager is leaving, but I believe that is not a result of the changes. She is leaving to be with her family in California."

Caught by surprise and a little sad, Duke slowly responded, "I like Mishka - I did not know."

Then Duke paused a while, staring into the fireplace that was burning bright. Maxx had just finished poking at it to get it going again.

"Unfortunately, I don't see employee changes and turnover. The breakdowns and system failures, well, I try to leave that to my operations director and human resources."

Maxx, as honest and straightforward but gentle as he always is, follows up, "Well, it's not only the turnover. That's not the heart of it. Duke, you know that I look at the business from a different lens than most other people. I see things from a 30,000-foot perspective. And from my perspective, it appears that things in your company are not going well. Duke, be honest with me, I am your brother, and I love you and care for you and your company. What's going on?"

Duke paused again... "um"... and then shaking his head, and then another, "um."

He wanted to be honest and upfront but was ashamed. But this was Maxx, and deep down, he knew that Maxx was always by Dukes' side. If anyone, Maxx could help.

"Well, there has been a lot of turnover in staff and management. And it appears to be trickling down with insecurities into the front-line staff. And I get that. I think?"

Maxx adds, "Well, look at it this way. Maggie is in the care of your company. If she is not getting the care she deserves, then how are the people being served who are not related to you?".

Duke straightened up in his chair, pushed his unfinished pastry aside, and paused.

"OK, I know that you are a no-excuses guy. Let me put this straight."

Pausing again... then looking right at Maxx.

"It seems that my managers are not happy. There are never-ending complaints in the office about other people and the regulations on audits, compliance, and insurance..."

Duke looked away from Maxx and looks down for a moment.

"They have taken over my focus and energy. It's hard, and I don't know what to do. We can't keep staff, and I am not sure why. I can't put my finger on it, and I don't feel that my managers are honest with me. I am stuck in this downward spiral, some kind of an out-of-control whirlwind."

Duke looked up at Maxx, and then down, and then up one more time.

"Do you think you can help the company and me? And Maggie?"

"Well, if you recall, at our lunch at the beginning of the year, I stated that I was picky about my clients and that I only take clients that are committed to change. It seems to me you are in a hurting place and need to make a change. Am I correct?"

"Yes, I think so."

"You think so?" Maxx confidently but slowly growled.

Just then, Duke stood up fast. And in a firm and committed voice,

"No, No... I mean yes, a big yes! I know so!"

"Good, then I will help you out, and we will make this work together. This is not the best place to talk, it's late, and we are tired. Let's say we meet at my house, in two weeks, Saturday. We can talk and come up with a plan to get you moving in a positive direction."

"In the meantime, read "Good to Great" again before you come. I need you to have the right mindset. Think about the two or three top problems that you are facing, you, the Duke, the CEO, not the company. And be prepared to bring a big box of crayons."

"Crayons?"

"Yes, a big box."

"OK, if you say so, I trust you!"

Weekend With Maxx

Two weeks later, Saturday at Maxx's home.

"Come on in, Duke. How are you today? Are you ready?"

"I am doing great, and yes, I am ready, cleared my calendar, and have turned my phone off. I have my number two guy who I can trust on call all weekend so we can focus."

"Good to hear, great!"

"So let's get started, coffee?"

"Sure."

"Hey, Maxx, I brought some answers to the questions you asked me, and I also brought a big box of crayons. Can't wait to find out what that's all about."

"Well, there something there that we need to explore. We can save that for later, though. Right now, let's keep an open mind.

Fill it?"

"Leave room for milk, please. Yup, that's it... thanks."

"So I would like you to think of me as a consultant, hired by you - personally, not your company. My goal is to help you become a better leader. We can work on management some other time. We can then center on the issues within your company. Most importantly, this is the tough part - don't think of me as the brother who called you 'the Duke'ster.' OK?"

"Not fair, Maxx! That's like asking someone not to think of the color red. Now that you mentioned it, I can't help but think 'the Duke'ster'."

The laughter broke the tension and eased the conversation as Maxx began...

"Let's get started. I asked you to take some strengths and gifts assessments over the week, and I have a good idea of what your personality is like, but I would like to hear what you think. When it comes to your leadership, what thoughts come to mind?"

Duke began, "To start, I never trained to be a leader. And I don't feel like someone can get an education in leadership. That is when it becomes more about skills."

Maxx adds, "My focus is on servant leadership; a compassionate heart in service to others. From the heart comes a strong foundation of leadership, and you can't fake it, and I truly believe this with all of my being. Everyone with a heartbeat can be a leader because everyone can influence at least one if not many people."

"Heartbeat, interesting.", Duke pondered. "As you know, I worked myself up the corporate ladder. I work well with people and get along with everyone... always a good team player. I think my biggest challenge is thinking daily. I mean, thinking of the big picture, as opposed to what I have to do next. There is always a fire to put out, always someone or something that needs to be managed or directed. And I find myself being sucked into a vortex, especially over the last six months, maybe more, and I can't get out of it.

"Go on," urged Maxx.

"I have trouble getting out from behind the desk, and like I said, seeing the big picture. I know I should, I want to, but I feel pressure to put out the fires. Sorry if that's repetitive."

"No, actually, it's perfect. Keep going, and don't edit yourself. Let yourself go and say what you feel."

"Well, OK, I feel like... well, I won't say this to anyone but you, Maxx. But I feel like a failure, and I am ashamed. I feel like the business is going down, and I won't be able to get out. I hire warm bodies just to fill in the seats. If you have a pulse, it almost guarantees you will get a job. I did a poor job in hiring managers and my number two and three executives. They're good, but not great, and..."

Duke pauses...

"Yes, and...?," blurts Maxx. "I am listening."

"They are followers and task-oriented like me. I hired mirror images of myself. And I think they follow my anxiety, practices, and well, I think my recent lack of confidence."

"Seems like an easy fix to me... go on."

"Really? Well, OK?"

Duke squirms around in his seat, making it look like he is trying to get comfortable in the chair when he is actually uncomfortable with the conversation. But he knows he must move on.

"I think if I can get a hold of a vision, stick to it daily. If I can get my number two and three to buy into it, and focus on the future, then I think we can get out of this hole I put us in."

Over the next several hours, Maxx invested time into Duke's personality, life, and divorce last year. They talked about Duke moving back to Brooklyn from Staten Island, which according to Duke, "the divorce was a much bigger blow to my ego and a negative boost to my anxiety level than I realized. It knocked me down for a long time, and I didn't know it - I think I am still down and out."

Together, Maxx and Duke had some emotional moments as well, especially in the care of Maggie. Duke felt like the business kept him away from Maggie. "Ironic," as Duke put it, "since my business is all about caring for her."

"Let's make some lunch. I bought some nice fresh rolls and a bunch of cold cuts. Ham, salami, capicola, provolone, red peppers, nice red tomatoes, and wait for it, wait for it...."

Excited for Duke, Maxx blurts out, "Zeppoles!"

"Wow, Maxx, you are great. It almost brought a tear to my eye. The left one, I think. We used to do these kinds of lunches all the time. Did I say, Wow!"

"Maxx, before we eat, I want to say one thing. Our talk was great, and it was over three hours. It seemed like 15 minutes. I didn't realize how important talking these things out is for me. I would guess for anyone who runs a company, the isolation factor sneaks in. Getting it out was cathartic and freeing. I feel like a boulder has been lifted off my shoulder. And we didn't even start talking about the business, yet."

Maxx followed up, "Something that I believe you need is a mastermind group. There you can talk with others regularly and get good honest feedback. I will give you information on mastermind groups later. This afternoon, we will talk about the business, but I think I already know the plan. I just need one thing from you."

"What's that?"

"The vision."

"Wait, I thought you were going to help me with that part."

"I will help you in the process of executing the vision, but it's your business, you are the leader, it must be your vision - not mine. Don't worry, I already see it in you - you just have to let it out."

"You know, before I forget - this whole servant leadership thing - I like the way it sounds."

"Yup, you have it in you - I see it as a brand-new day.", Maxx added with a spark in his voice. "You are like Captain America, yet you don't know it yet. Once you realize your powers, you will be able to do wonderful and great things for a boatload of people."

"Eat Duke! I still need more info from you, but first, eat! And save me a Zep."

Three Seconds to Vision

"Those Zeppoles were good. Now a cup of espresso would be nice."

"Coming up, Duke."

"Wait - slow down. You have an espresso machine?"

"Just bought it last month; I love it. It makes some good foam, too. Here 'ya go."

"Duke, you are aware that running a healthcare business that is home care and hospice at the same time is unique. There are some out there but still not very common. I see it as the wave of the future.

The businesses are similar on the front line in caring for the families and patients. So, I would expect that's what made you love the company as you were moving up the ladder."

"Yup, but I learned it is the clinical side that is a bit different and more challenging than I thought. That with the combined compliance, insurance, and all the regulatory work is intensive. I understand it's a system of checks and balances and required...

But it's turning out to be the driving force of the business."

"Yes, you are correct on all counts. However, just because other healthcare organizations are compliance-focused does not mean that the vision cannot be centered and people-focused.

Most organizations have a stated vision where the middle management and the front-line staff have no idea what it is. They're driven by the fires that they feel need to be put out. The fires are the smallest priorities that scream out at them every day. These very fires keep their focus away from the big picture.

They have trouble discerning on a minute to minute, day to day basis, the important versus the priority. For you, Duke, you are a priority-driven individual, and that is good, but it's going to be your biggest challenge. You must focus on what's important.

OK, tell me more - start with the top down. Talk about each of your executives, then directors, and managers of each region. Remember, I am in the information collecting mode here, so keep talking, and I will guide you. The answers will come later - much later."

"Well, we have the Chief Operations Officer, Joe..."

Dinner Time

"It's 5:15 p.m. We have been talking all day. I need to fill in some gaps, but I fill them in over the next few weeks. I've got to do some research. Then I'm going to bring together the beginnings of a plan. I already have a good idea of the points that we should focus on, and I can give them to you in a week. The bigger plan will come later.

So, let's make dinner and talk about some other stuff. Like your new home."

"Sounds good, Maxx. What's for dinner?"

"Well, you are going to help me make it. Good old fashioned, handmade hamburgers and fries."

"Nice - just like the good 'old days. What do you want me to do?"

"Grab those red potatoes, clean them, and slice them up just like the way we used to do it with Ginger and Maggie, mom and dad."

"Skin and all, right?"

"Yup!"

"So, I purposely saved the most important topic for now, while we are prepping for dinner. I wanted your mind to be in a good place after you released all that information from what was bothering you and holding you back."

Maxx had just dropped an egg into the chopped meat and started to mix all the ingredients with his hands. Duke finished washing the potatoes.

"OK, but first, where's the cutting board?"

"Second drawer down, and to the right."

"Got it! OK, shoot!"

"Duke, listen to me carefully. I will ask you a question, and I want you to answer me as quickly as possible. Don't think too long about it - OK?"

"OK?"

"You have three seconds, and I am going to count.

Think about your business 20 years from now. You are celebrating a successful year. Your company has tripled in size, you have partnered with some other organizations, you and the business are well known. You are a speaker and consultant for other executives and professional organizations."

"Sounds good..."

"You are now at a ceremony that you prepared for your employees - all 1,500 of them and their significant others. It's a huge gathering. You are giving out awards to those people who excelled - and I know you, Duke, you love giving out awards."

"Yup, I love appreciating others. I think that was the problem with where I am now...."

"Stop - Duke, don't come back to now. Go back to giving out the awards."

Maxx is just finishing the third burger and placing it on the plate.

"Darn, I forgot to turn on the barbecue. Hold on!"

Duke singing, "Giving out the awards to people,

giving out the awards,

giving out the awards to people,

giving out the awards."

"I am back. Are you with me?"

"Yes, and enjoying the process."

"So you are about to give out the awards, and you are giving a speech, a short one but one that shows your sincere appreciation and gratitude for the hardworking people of your organization. And you talk about fulfilling the daily mission by always keeping the vision alive and well."

"Duke, in as few words as possible - what is that vision?"

"OH, that's easy - Maggie!"

"Huh? OK, Duke, that's not what I was expecting."

"Well, it has to do with Maggie. I was thinking about this all day, and I would like us to become a dementia centered organization - not exclusively dementia but the 'go-to' organization. An organization that will be known for its care, education, and support of those diagnosed with dementia, their families, and the community. Yup, definitely in the community."

"Well, that's good - more focused than it was before. We have to fine-tune it, but it has heart and meaning behind it - it has a story behind it, and you can easily keep it alive with the help of Maggie."

"Who would have thought that Maggie would be the start of the vision of your company.

Duke, let's fill up and eat dessert!"

Dessert

"I can't believe you made that cheesecake. It was thick and creamy. And being outside, it's peaceful and quiet, with a nice crackling fire. Thanks, Maxx - this is the perfect end to a day that I hope will bring much more like it."

"My pleasure, I like baking, but I don't do it too much. I must say I enjoyed the day, too. Even though I started by asking you not to think of me as your brother but your consultant, it wasn't like that for me. I felt like we were brothers again. I hope we can do this more often - even if it's for business."

"I have to be honest; it was the same with me. I never thought of you as my consultant. It was hard for me to see you beyond my older brother. Still, now, after guiding me through that process and teaching me about strategic planning and how the culture and subcultures of the business need to change, well, I was impressed, really, really impressed. So now, when it comes to our roles together, I think I can easily make the switch from consultant to brother and back."

"That's good - really good. Now, let's see what happens if I add some more wood to that fire."

Follow Up Meeting

It's the holiday season in December, almost six weeks after Duke and Maxx had their burgers, cheesecake, and 'talk.' Maxx has researched the home care and hospice business and naturally added the assisted living business as well. "It's all connected and harmonious," he said.

Maxx wanted to meet with Duke face to face on several occasions, but the 'Sunshine Dementia' contract in Florida took up a lot of his time. He was also enjoying the nice warm weather and was considering purchasing a condo near Miami. Yet, he knew that he had to honor his commitment to Duke, his leadership, and his company. So, Maxx contacted Duke on Christmas Day to wish him God's blessings and make an appointment to invest the day together, the day after New Year's, January 2, 2019.

"It's time to propose the 'Maggie plan'," Maxx exclaimed, leaving Duke in another optimistically curious state.

"Hey, Maxx, we never discussed the box of crayons."

"Oh, that's one of the **'Seven Strategies'** outline I have for you. We'll talk about it for sure! Hey, Be safe, and God Bless You. I have to call Maggie and Ginger now. See you on January 2 at my place. Goodbye, Duke, and Merry Christmas."

Maxx calls Ginger and wishes her the best, giving all his love and God's blessings. But Maggie isn't doing well.

The last full sentence Maggie said was when Maxx and Ginger were together with Maggie. The time when Maggie repeated, "What am I doing here? What am I doing here?"

Ginger sadly stated, "As time went on, those words became more and more garbled, whereas by the time of Thanksgiving, she stopped talking completely. Now she stares, and we can't get her out of bed. She mostly stays in the fetal position unless we prop her up, so she is comfortable eating."

Maxx, it's so sad to watch every day. I am slowly watching my sister and best friend wither away into nothingness."

"Ginger, I am so sorry. I can't imagine how hard this is for you. She is your best friend. I wish I were there to hold you, sis."

"Sis? You haven't called me that in years, many years. I like it. It makes me feel good, connected, and loved."

"OK, then sis' it is.! Hey, I am flying up before New Year's, maybe New Year's eve. I will come by, and we can get together for the evening. Does that sound good to you? We can bang pots and pans like we did when we were kids at 9 p.m. and then go to bed."

"I remember we used to do that every year. But Maggie was in charge. She took care of all the stuff. It was her thing."

"It can still be her thing. It will be her thing. I am excited."

"Me too! Maxx!"

"Great, OK, I will see you on New Year's Eve. I will let you know when my flight arrives, and we can set a time. God Bless You, Ginger! God Bless You! And God Bless Maggie!"

New Year's Eve

Maxx, Duke, Ginger, and Maggie all had a good time. Cooking and talking, reminiscing, and laughing. And when it came time, 9 p.m., to bang the pots and pans, everyone held onto something to knock together. Even Maggie had two small spoons to hold. And they counted down and banged away, and Maggie smiled. The first time showing any emotion in over a month - and Ginger cried, and Maxx cried, and Duke cried too.

It's January 2nd, Maxx is waiting for Duke to knock on the door. Maxx prepared a nice breakfast with bagels, lox, walnuts-raisin cream cheese, and Duke's favorite cream cheese with onions and chives.

Duke was supposed to come by at 9 a.m., but it's now 10 a.m.

"Good thing I didn't cook," Maxx thought. "Well, I will give him the benefit of the doubt. I can always make a fresh pot of coffee." Just then, Maxx'x phone began to sing the tune, **'What a Wonderful World'**. The ID of the caller showed that it was Duke.

"Hey, brother, good morning. Are you OK?"

"Sorry, sorry, Maxx. So sorry, I did not call you earlier. My number two, my vice president, just died this morning. I am at his home now with his family. We are going to have to postpone our meeting. I will get back to you in a few days."

"Take care of things, Duke. So sorry, please express my condolences to the family and you, of course. I know the two of you were close and working together for a long time."

"Thanks, Maxx - Take care."

March 14: Two and a half months later - Duke makes an appointment with Maxx.

"Happy St. Patrick's Day! Maxx, it's been crazy. I don't recall ever having to work so hard. I slept in my office, on the floor, many nights. We haven't caught up yet. And just when we started the process of interviewing for the new number two, I realized that it might be important that you and I have that meeting."

"Good to hear from you and Happy St. Pats, too, and a good idea. Before you hire anyone, you might want to hear what I have to say. Some of the advice might be crucial in making your decisions in hiring. I would suggest to keep collecting resumes and put everything on hold for 30 days. Can you do that?"

"Yes, I think so. How does next weekend sound."

"I will be heading down to Florida to finish up some loose ends with "Sunshine Dementia, and coming home Sunday afternoon. So that won't work. Let's do April 5. I am free the whole day, and we can talk?"

"OK, done deal - April 5. Maxx, this time, I will bring bagels and cream cheese."

"Don't forget the lox. See you then - 8 a.m. sharp, April 5."

Chapter Four – The Maggie Plan

April 5th

Duke was able to put out the many fires after his long-time work companion and the chief operating officer died on January 2. This event put Maxx's plans of introducing his seven strategies on hold. Through it all, and with Maxx's help, Duke maintained his optimism and looked forward to Maxx's proposals. Duke was eagerly anticipating changing the company around, and he was also looking forward to the bagels.

"I have bagels, lox, and cream cheese. Still fresh and hot. How are you, Maxx?"

"Doing great, Duke, doing great! How are you holding up? You had a rough few months, and I can only imagine the waters are still a bit choppy. Talk to me."

Here, put those bagels on this plate. I'll get the utensils."

"Yeah, it's been rough, but I think things are starting to level off. Don't get me wrong, there is still a mess of stuff to get in order, and the little fires we have to put out daily are still there. Our firemen are scattered, the staff is all over the place trying to make amends, and always in catch-up mode. Maxx, it seems like we are always one step forward and two steps back. I don't even know where we are financially. I'm still trying to get a hold of the daily operations. That's why I am looking forward to hearing what your view is. I have three, maybe four individuals lined up for the chief operating officer's position, but wanted to wait."

"Here's some fresh-squeezed orange juice and the butter since the bagels are still hot. You know we love our melted butter on the soft hot bagels."

"We used to call them 'Brooklyn sauteed bagels in butter.' Not sure why we called them sauteed, but hey, we were kids then and had fun. Those were the good old days. I would love to go back to those days, just for a few hours. Our biggest worry was trying to get enough guys to have a decent stick ball game."

Maxx agreed, "Stick-ball in the summer in New York! Now, that's a memory. And we would play for hours, non-stop..."

"Except when the ice cream truck came around. It was the only time we rested. We wouldn't even stop to use the restroom."

"You know, I never realized that. Interesting..."

"And then, mom would yell out the door at dinner time to call us in for dinner. I miss mom..."

"Speaking of interesting, hmm... I miss mom too."

Taking charge, Maxx yelled, "OK, let's get to business here. We have much to discuss."

"OK." said Duke, "but first, can you please pass the cream cheese and the bagels? Please!"

"Duke, I did a lot of research. Locally, nationally and across the globe. It seems that well, this dementia problem is growing, slowly but growing, and there is no slow down predicted. Drug companies have pulled out of any cure. The drugs that are out there are only fooling people by masking the symptoms, only to lead people to the false hope that the drugs slow down the disease."

"Yes, I know... not a lot of people know that, and unfortunately, they start learning when it's too late."

"Correct, and it appears to me that there is an over-abundance of caregiver info, and I mean a lot, and rightfully so. Plenty of groups, consultants, and coaches to help families get through the process, whether it be understanding the medical and clinical side, the insurance side, medical billing, or coping with and the 'how-to's' on dealing with the day-to-day struggles of care.

Duke - there is a ton of information out there to the point that it's difficult to find an expert in the field. Yet, they are all so-called experts. It's a challenging field of stalkers taking prey on the uneducated and uninformed."

"I do understand. I'm listening," says Duke as he is polishing off the second half of his second bagel. "By the way, this orange juice is really good!"

"Thanks, Duke. So keep in mind, I was looking into the business side of healthcare back in January when we were supposed to meet. Since we didn't meet, I kept researching and learning, researching, and learning. I discovered something interesting. I will mention it now but will talk in detail later.

I noticed these companies: the assisted living, home care, and hospice organizations. I have researched their marketing and advertising to understand how they cater to the dementia population. They generalize that they serve the dementia population but offer no technical information. It's not focused on dementia. It's like a coffee house saying they serve the best coffee in the world. Just because they say it doesn't mean it is the best."

"Wait a minute - What do you mean?"

"Well, they say they specialize and don't. I looked deeper into many of these companies, made phone calls, and even visited, but they don't do anything special - nothing. Duke, I find this disturbing and heartbreaking because the families and patients don't know what to look for beyond the empty facade.

Oh! Maybe they have a separate building or section of a building. Or perhaps they might have a director who attended a dementia class or a nurse that worked in dementia her whole career, but that's it.

Duke, this is all over, the United States anyway, from what I can tell. There are exceptions, of course. Duke, your company, does state that it caters to the dementia population, but it also states that it serves dementia patients and families alongside other diseases and illnesses."

"That's right, well, I guess it does. I haven't looked at our marketing materials in a while. Are you saying that is wrong?"

"Yes, at least morally wrong."

"The challenge is that organizations state that they specialize and don't. That leaves you wide open to the market. There are no or little checks and balances to tell the people on the important items. Some state organizations have regulations that dictate that if an organization says it is a dementia care facility, the staff must be trained. But what does 'train' mean?

And that's where I think you can specialize with a high-end, world-class training and certification program within a dementia care system. One that will bring your front-line staff, your support staff, and all your managers and directors to the same high competency level to best serve the patient and family.

Duke - this could bring your organization to the highest level of integrity possible."

After swallowing his last bite, Duke takes notes, his first set of notes for the day. As he writes, he whispers, "five-star, world-class...." And what was that you said about integrity. Oh, wait, "highest level of integrity."

"So, why did you write that down, Duke?"

Duke stared right at Maxx... "It's a dream that I just turned into a reality and will make it a goal!"

"Excellent, Duke! Now we are moving forward... so let me explain further.

Specialize, fine-tune your niche! We talked about this in your vision. Be a dementia-based organization. Live, breathe, eat, drink, and sleep dementia and share everything with everyone. Become the go-to; when people think of dementia, they should think of your company. I want you to be the leader of a Dementia Friendly Facility™. Become associated with a learning system that serves you and your employees by assessing, training, and certifying your organization. Become a learning organization that can transform dementia care.

Think butterfly, Duke."

Hey, you heard of 'Band-aids' right, or 'Q-tips'? Well, those are brand names referring to adhesive bandages and cotton swabs. You eventually want the same thing - at least in the region that you serve. You want doctors, nurses, hospitals, assisted living centers, nursing centers, clinics, adult day care centers, and anything else healthcare to think of your company when the word dementia pops up. It's called top-of-mind awareness or TOMA.

It will take some time, and it will take strong leadership, good marketing, ongoing training and development, and Duke, you can get it done. You need a good vision and, dare I say again, strong leadership. You need servant leadership - leadership that serves the people first."

"Hold on, Maxx. You mentioned butterfly. What do you mean?".

"Duke, it is theorized that the small breeze from butterfly wings can have a huge effect on situations on the other side of the world. It's only a theory, and I think it was proved by a bunch of college students. Anyhow, the meaning behind it is that small increments on a daily basis can have a big change in your business later on.

I use this saying frequently, 'Butterflies and elephants.'"

"Elephants? What is this with creatures and leadership?"

"More on that later, Duke."

Pet Peeves

"Something else that I find bothersome. Keeping in mind that in today's technology and internet world, the website and social media have become the main source of awareness for an organization's business - it's their storefront. Well, they hide their vision in the 'about' section. They don't post their leaders, or executive teams, or the people in the regions. Many sites are clinical or, at the other end, try not to be clinical by posting pictures of staff caring for older people, with clinical wording. It seems all template driven. Sorry, I digress, that's a pet peeve, and I shouldn't focus on it now. That's a job for your marketing team."

"Pass that orange juice, would 'ya? Please!"

"So, let me throw something else out there at you. And it comes as a result of the additional research I did between January and now. Dementia is climbing at a steady rate to increase by almost 400% by 2050. Cut that in half; that's 200% by 2035. Maybe those numbers are not exact but being exact is not important here. It gives us a feeling and understanding of what's happening. The population of the baby boomers is increasing as well. Some call the baby boomer population increase the 'Silver Tsunami.' Not sure how accurate that is, but for us, it's relevant.

The projected increase in dementia reflects that number. The number of elderly patients cared for by their children as primary caregivers at home is also steadily increasing.

The home care business is increasing steadily with the increase in dementia patients. I haven't looked at the numbers, but I bet the growth is the same or at least a bit higher if you chart it out.

Of course, hospice care is increasing as well.

Currently, the number of dementia patients receiving home-care, nationally, is somewhere near 35%. Today, the top numbers of those cancer and heart patients - and those numbers are declining each year.

Duke - can you see what's happening?

Boomers are increasing, and dementia is rising. Combine those numbers, and you have an alarming increase in dementia care that is needed. Duke, I don't think the United States is ready. At least they don't look like they are preparing."

"Yes, Maxx, those numbers I do know about, and I do not think my company is in a place to grow. We are in the same place we were five years ago. Our hospice side has not grown at all."

"I understand, Duke. I am sure you know that the hospice percentages are even higher. I think it was 40-45% are dementia patients nationally. And here is where I started noticing this open hole in the business.

I researched and looked at home-care, hospice, and assisted living centers, and it was the same across the board. Very few, and I mean less than 10% of the companies I could find, specialize in dementia care.

My criteria: I was looking at 100% or close to all staff trained and certified, with ongoing training. And most of the staff had to be experienced with at least 3-7 years. These organizations were up to date on proper living conditions, lighting, appropriate activities, scheduling, and dining arrangements. By the way, I found it to be very important, limiting the sundowning practices, and more. There is a large list of items an organization can put into practice. A full service, world-class dementia organization only needs a well-trained staff, at least to start. A more knowledgeable staff will have the foundation to better care for the patients. Here is where knowledge equals power or the power to serve."

"OK, Duke, you listening?

I could be off, remember that's my research, but even if I'm off, let's say by 30 percent, that means 6-7 out of 10 companies do not specialize in the market they're in now. To be clear, what I mean by specializing is that they don't 'walk the talk'.

I will give you three examples of some research I did; one hospice, one home-care, and one assisted living. I called and visited each, asking questions face to face, researched their companies and websites.

The hospice and home-care were very similar. They both advertised that they care for dementia patients and their families, hinting that they offer dementia care as a specialty. Yet, there was no talk or marketing on whether anyone has the experience, training, or certification. When I asked both companies, they could not provide an answer. They had nothing to say. Now I am not saying that they were not experienced or trained, but nowhere did I find any confidence in the communication. For me, no confidence equals no vision, which equals no leadership, although the management might have been good; however, there is no leadership."

"OK, so now the assisted living centers. I went to three places that advertised that they have a separate dementia center, unit, or building. They marketed that they cared for dementia patients, with the impression that they specialized in this service. Not one of them had a dementia certification or geriatric care license, or degree, or anything. They may well have mentioned that an employee or two have worked for the company for five or seven years or anything like that but not so much more than that minimum because it is just enough to get by for them. This brings me to another point! Turnover is very high in all these places."

Duke added, "Tell me about it; I can't keep people. They leave for 50 cents or a dollar more an hour. It's crazy."

"Duke, with the proposal I have for you, your turnover should be low. Remember, your focus is on your leadership and the vision, not compliance, and not the fires. They are important, but not your focus. Those issues will be someone else's job. Your job will be to serve your company by serving your people."

"OK, enough of me talking about generalities. Let me introduce this to you. Let's call it 'The Maggie Formula' for now.

The first section is on Attitude; Your attitude.
Duke, you must possess the attitude of the servant leader.

The second section is three areas of focus:

Leadership, Marketing, Training & Development.

The third section is 'Seven Leadership Strategies'.

"We have talked about the leadership and the vision at length. We will get into detail later, but in essence, you need to know your new vision; with all your heart, mind, and soul. Moreover, your new vision is your drive. As you work on your drive to fulfill the vision, you will find your passion.

You need to establish a significant buy-in from your leadership team before you can move forward. Since you are currently hiring a chief operating officer, getting their buy-in will be a big first step that cannot be avoided. You can't move to step two unless your team is with you 110%."

Dementia Friendly Facility™

"Got it so far, Duke?"

"So far, I do. There is an untapped niche in the dementia field. Well, it's tapped, but only a few organizations are in and not the way I think you want me to go. The home care, hospice, and assisted living centers are not exactly who they are or who they say they are. As the incidents with dementia are increasing, the population is rising, and then the consumer will get smarter.

And I'm sort of feeling like the consumer isn't necessarily the family caregivers or the patients themselves. It's a lot bigger.

As far as putting my employees first, I don't want to say it. I want to do it; more significantly, I am going to need help there. Probably in creating a doable action plan and be held accountable. That's my hard part, which is getting into long-term thinking, stop putting out fires, and well, burn my micro-management hat.

But I can see that happening. I understand that there will always be fires in the people business I am in, but that doesn't mean I have to put them out. The mayor of New York doesn't put out the fires in Brooklyn. A designated group of experienced, educated people dedicated to that mission is charged with that work. I know it, now, to do that - well, that's something I need to work on."

"Duke, that will be 90% of the first step. If you can get that part, I think much of the rest will follow. That's why the first step in the plan is your attitude. Suppose you start to look at each step, one step at a time. See problems as challenges; you will be able to overcome them and move forward. Instead of one step forward and two back, you will move two steps forward and maybe one back but still moving forward. In 5-10 years, you will be well-positioned in the market as the only Dementia Friendly Facility™ and organization in the region."

Now let's get back to the formula.

As I stated, the first area is the leader's attitude, including the vision. The vision will need a full strategic plan, but if it's broken down into small pieces, it will be manageable so that you can cast it to everyone you meet."

"And number two, Maxx?"

"Two represents three areas of focus, especially when it comes to collaboration and designation of specific duties; Leadership, Marketing, and Training & Development. These areas all require their own vision and mission, which are connected to the vision of the organization.

It will require you to tap into the leadership that we have cultivated in step one, which is the leadership and management that is willing to share and collaborate with the organization. We are looking for gifted people with strengths in specific areas: no silos or lone wolves.

Oh, that's another big pet peeve of mine. There are people, teams working in silos as a result of the structure or the way of doing business. Some people develop a lone wolf mentality, as well. It's the ones that come into this business as lone wolves that you need to watch for... but I digress - sorry. We will talk more about that later."

In agreement, Duke showed his understanding, "Silos and lone wolves, I can see that. People working on their own, in their bubble with their plan. But Maxx, I don't see that as their fault. Many of my employees work alone and don't see other team members for weeks sometimes."

"Duke, I understand and appreciate that. Remember, as a consultant, I work alone and travel alone but can still collaborate and share. With your company, you're going to have to do this yourself and let people see that sharing is crucial even if they're working alone. They can still have that team attitude. It's the lone wolves that I am most concerned about - more on that later."

"OK, Maxx, how about I clean up before moving on. I will make a fresh pot of coffee."

"That's a good idea."

"Maxx, you are running out of cream. We have enough for today, but not sure if you will have enough for the next few days."

"Thanks, I was planning on shopping tomorrow. I have to for Ginger and Maggie anyhow. But thanks again."

"Here's a fresh cup for you. So let me hear about areas two and three; Marketing, and then Training & Development."

"Marketing is, of course, a broad topic, and I forget how many areas I discuss in the report I have for you, but it's far-reaching and deep. It covers areas as small as memory cafe, dementia support groups, church collaboration, special hubs for communicating with doctors and nurses, researchers and schools, writing articles, and public speaking.

The two operative words for this transformation will be 'share' and 'collaboration.' The leadership and, specifically, the marketing department's leadership and management must collaborate with the training and development. It's a marriage.

The marketing role is not to make the sale but to get the information in front of the people, including professionals, or caregivers or patients, or the community. They must address the type of information, the quality of the information, and the transmission of that information, and the ability to make it easy to assimilate. "

"Then, of course, training and development or as you put it T&D. Which should also include research as part of the department's duties. They should be the certifying body of the company that will certify every first line and second line staff in dementia. The team at Wellspring Senior Care will help you become a certified Dementia Friendly Facility™. They do all the research, training, and certification - an excellent accountability system which is a major asset.

As you already know, accountability is a key element in increasing the significance and the individual's value, and skill levels. Your employees will behave with a higher level of integrity. And that directly correlates to what you wrote down earlier, turning your dream into a reality.

So back to where we were.

Additionally, there should be an internal certification for those who want to learn and do more. This is important, a dementia support certification for all office staff and those who do not deal with dementia patients first hand. Everyone, and I mean, everyone, should have a basic understanding of dementia.

Again, there is a collaboration required with the Marketing and Training & Development departments. As I said earlier, the Wellspring Senior Care company can help you become a certified Dementia Friendly Facility™.

And Duke, it takes time. With the number of employees you have, spread out over several states, it will take a couple of years to get everyone trained and certified. But once your turnover decreases, your investment in training will become manageable, and by that time, you should be confident and certified as a Dementia Friendly Facility™."

'So, Duke, are you listening?"

'Yes, of course, Maxx."

"Sorry, Duke, I was being facetious. Every one of your staff is an advertisement for your company. And if you are doing a good job, wait no, a great job in serving your employees, they will want to talk about you and your company's services. Certifying them provides an immense portion of the information they need to talk about you - naturally and confidently, instead of being forced into a checklist that we may see within the sales program.

And, with the 'live certification program,' the office staff will have a higher appreciation for the front-line teams caring for the patients and families."

"Wait, Maxx, 'live certification program'? You didn't mention that earlier."

"That's the training, certification, and accountability program Wellspring Senior Care implements. In essence, it's life because it's ongoing, regular, and consistent. You have heard of Kaizen, haven't you, Duke?"

"Kaizen, yes. But isn't that some kind of production efficiency program from Japan?"

"Well, yes Duke, in a way. But it's much more than that. I address it in the seven strategies. But it's something you should consider. I like to look at it as a philosophy and mindset. I like what Wellspring is doing; that's why I pointed it out."

"So it's like, every day, giving the seeds the right soil and water and access to the right sunlight so growth can occur naturally over time. So, it's life!"

"Correct, Duke. That's a nice way of putting it, and you should use that as an analogy for your visions presentations."

"OK, Maxx, let me write that down..."

Introducing The Seven Strategies

"Okay Duke, let's move forward to the seven strategies or, as I like to call them, the touchpoints. If it's OK with you, I will glance over them as there is more detail than we have time. Let's agree to save the detail for discussion after today. Is that OK with you, Duke?"

"Sounds good, Maxx. Hey, you got my mind racing, and it needs to slow down. It's one o'clock. We have been at this for over four hours. How about we break? I will order pizza from Lenny and John's. Sounds good?"

"Best idea today, Duke!"

"Pepperoni?"

"Olives too, please, and onions?"

"You got it!"

Maxx and Duke intentionally take a break and talk about Maggie and how they will be a bigger part of her care from now on.

"Maxx, after we finish talking, let's go visit Magmore's significant Ginger. Let's break around 4 p.m."

"Good idea; I think Ginger might need some emotional and spiritual support. She seems to have been down the past few days. She has been more sad than usual."

"I agree. The caregiver gives a good amount of support, and she is wonderful, but Ginger needs us to hold her up as well. OK, it's agreed. Four o'clock."

"So, we talked about leadership, marketing and research," as Maxx rebooted the conversation. Maxx moved on to review and added a few more concepts, and answered questions from Duke. About an hour later...

"Now let me share the seven strategies; these are areas that are important to practice daily and are what I believe will be inherently important to your success in the business of dementia as a specialty and praxis. Duke, I truly believe that these seven strategies, and let me add these are only seven of many, but the seven strategies, if followed, could make you a world-class operation. You will be able to lead with integrity and confidence. You and your staff, guaranteed."

"Praxis, I heard that before. Remind me..."

"Praxis, for me, in your situation is a broader and higher-level word than practice. You hear doctors say that "they practice medicine." Well, praxis is engaging, applying, exercising, realizing, or practicing ideas. The practice is the practical application of the praxis - which I would say is the skill. So, what you are doing today is learning new concepts and skills. You will grow and develop those ideas and skills, teach, coach, and mentor others who will, in turn, do the same. It's like disciplining others. And those skills, ideas get realized and applied daily. That's praxis - it's more of a strategic view as the practice is more of a tactical notion."

"Duke, I like to use 'learning' and 'praxis' as I believe they are words that are inherently involved in the principles of servant leadership. They both require a synergy. They refer to systems as opposed to programs. For me, they are relationship-based."

"Got it...! Maxx."

"As you already know, the healthcare business is more challenging than ever before. There are assisted living, hospice, and home-care businesses opening up every day, each one undercutting the other or trying to manipulate the consumer into using their service. Insurance, regulations, shrinking margins, and the education level of the employee are all changing. And you must keep up with that change. If you are not changing, you are dying.

Duke, you want to take these seven strategies, touchpoints and apply them in every area of your life and make them applicable in the lives of others. You want to make them habits in your everyday routine.

I created a complete portfolio for you, explaining them in detail with examples, ideas, and talking points.

Here they are in a nutshell:

1. Passion
2. Chameleon
3. Vision
4. Kaizen
5. Effective
6. Empower
7. Tribe

These are the words used to explain a much bigger concept. We will have to put time aside to discuss the concepts in detail and understand how they apply to your business, especially if you want a strong foundation and focus on dementia care.

I want to add that many of your partners are assisted-living centers and partners in the patient's mutual service, yet not corporate partners. These seven strategies would apply to them, as well. And as part of the second step, you may want to seriously consider offering them some kind of complimentary support within the program. Talk to Wellspring Senior Care for ideas on how to collaborate with your partners. And, I have some deeper thoughts and ideas on that as well. When you do talk with them, let's share."

"Back to the strategies, you must encompass them in every aspect of your life and your business."

"The first is passion. You must be passionate about the needs of the patient and their families. Passionate about how you care for them. Making each area of what you and your organization do is better, faster, and more effective but might not be as efficient. Efficient could be a killer. Employees come first and are essential, but you must be well reminded that the patient is your priority. Your passion for the patient and their needs will create a fire in the passion for the employees. And no passion for employees means you cannot serve the customer well.

The second is the chameleon. You have to change and adapt by keeping your heart mostly on the patient, your pulse on the market, and your hands on your employees, your mind on finances and regulations. Your spirit must stay in the heart of the vision."

Duke blurted out, "Maxx, wait, my mind needs a break. Let me be still a moment."

"Sure, Duke. Sorry, my enthusiasm sometimes gets the best of me. I think some quiet and still time is good for both of us. Let me know when you are ready."

"Maxx, coffee?"

"No, thanks! I am good for the rest of the day. I could go for a Zeppole; any left?'"

"I will bring one in for you. Do you want me to nuke it in the microwave - 10 seconds?"

"That works - thanks!"

After Duke brought out his coffee and Zeppole for Maxx, they both sat down and were quiet. Yet, Duke's mind was racing in a hundred different directions.

"Duke, I want to add that with each strategy, there is an overlap. Each area will overlap, complimenting, and adding to one or all of the areas. To make them part of what you do, we have to separate them to distinguish and understand them, and when we step back, you will see each of these touchpoints are colors in a tapestry of the rainbow you will cast over your business and onto your employees."

"Are you ready to continue, Duke?"

"Well, not really... but go ahead. You can start as I finish this Zep."

"The third strategy, Kaizen, sometimes you will see it called CANI. I customize this a bit from the original Japanese philosophy. Kaizen is the ongoing, regular, and consistent development of the individual, the team, the tribe, and the employee; in the eyes of the leader."

"There are two ways to look at this but all the same action. In the leader's eyes, it's more of a strategic approach, wherein the employee's eyes are more tactical. As a leader, you need to understand both sides of that coin. Employees need to trust but not necessarily understand the leaders' side. This is where the 'live certification' concept was born by Wellspring Senior Care. It's also the heart of the Dementia Friendly Facility™ certification process."

"The fourth strategy is the vision. Need I say more. You must always motivate, inspire - walk the talk, talk about the vision and mission. You must sleep it, drink it, eat it, and breathe it. The vision must be in the DNA of your blood."

"Duke, what is the vision of your company? Don't answer that...

I wasn't going to include vision in this list because we talked about it in the prior section, but then I realized, well, it's that important. What reinforced my decision to include this was Maggie, and the last few sentences she spoke."

"Maggie? What do you mean? How could Maggie have convinced you?"

"Well, when Maggie had those two episodes where she repeated, "Who am I?' and 'What am I doing here?'. It made me think about how important it is to have that identity of who we are and our purpose. We all need to know who we are and why we are here. Not only in the organization where we work, but in life as well. The vision is a big part of answering that question. A bit more on that later. Time is running out."

"The fifth strategy is being effective as opposed to being efficient. It's about quality vs. quantity.

It's about the employee versus compliance or being bottom-line focused. It's about living the vision and how the company lives it on a daily basis.

The strategy is how the vision will take place, and for you, for the future of healthcare, I would emphatically state to be effective and focus on quality.

That does not mean that the numbers, compliance, and also the rules and regulations don't matter. They do matter and are important. But not the most important, and very seldom do they take priority over the patient and the employee."

"Second, from last, strategy six is empowerment. That's where the big box of crayons comes in. If you don't empower your employees, you don't and won't grow. I have seen that the business of micro-managing, which is a control and insecurity issue brought on by poor management, and ineffective leadership, crushes employees. It makes them stifle and stop, only performing at their minimum. From what little I can see from my vantage point - without a vision and an intentional strategy, compliance kills empowerment. Let me restate, the focus on compliance kills empowering your employees. More on the crayons later."

"Maxx, this is incredible. I feel like I have let my employees down. I focused on the bottom line and the regulations to stay in business that I never considered my employees.

Maxx - these are people with lives and families. And, I realized this earlier and have to talk it out, so I understand it better.

I invested so much time and energy into those things that do not produce a positive atmosphere. Instead of centering my attention on the employees. Maxx, I..."

Duke paused and was having trouble speaking. He cleared his throat, and...

"I don't know my employees."

"But you will! Duke, you will, and I will be here for you. Holding your hand and holding you up. Duke - are you OK?"

"Yup, I am good. Let's move on..."

"Last but not least, number seven is the Tribe. The tribe is at the heart of the matter, the vision. They are a cohesive, committed set of individuals who realize a higher-level function within the company.

Teams are focused on shared goals, but the values and the identity are not as important or may not be perceived as important by the leadership or management. The business you are in, the hospice and home care business and this may also be the same for assisted living, has a high propensity of individuals in teams or even groups that act as silos and lone wolves.

Groups and teams are less focused on their values and more concentrated on the 'getting things done at any cost' attitude. Like the other strategies, we will go over this in more detail."

Duke, keep in mind, these are not the end-all seven strategies. There are more, and as we start listing more, we will see a significant overlap. As we move into these seven, others will emerge, some consciously, others we may not see until later.

But this is where I see that the home care, hospice, and assisted living businesses need to start. These seven strategies are starting points and easy concepts where you, your C-level team, and your employees can easily understand and assimilate. It will take time, but it will work if you...."

Just then, a melody plays from Maxx's phone, "...under the boardwalk, boardwalk..."

"Hey, that's my phone."

"Love that tune, Maxx. Yeah, it reminds me of some of the good 'ole days..."

"Oh, it's Ginger... Hi Ginger!"

"Maxx, I think Maggie is gone... OK, Duke is with me. We are heading over right now. Did you call the nurse?"

"Yes, she is on the way."

"Good, we are leaving now and should be there in about 20 minutes."

"OK, see you then... you have the key, right?"

"Yes, we will come right in... is the aide with you?"

"Yes, she is cleaning Maggie up and making her decent."

"We are on the way."

The Funeral

Maggie died on the afternoon of April 5, the day Duke and Maxx were just finishing up their conversation. Ginger, Maxx, and Duke just began eating breakfast together a few days after Maggie's death. Duke was making and serving breakfast.

"How are you holding up, Ginger?"

"Better than I thought I would. Not so many eggs, and only one slice of bacon, please, Duke."

"Sure, Ginger. Did you sleep, OK?"

"Thanks, Duke. Can you pass the salt, too, please? Well, I didn't sleep well the night Maggie died, but I slept well for the past two nights. How about you two?"

"Well, I didn't sleep much, but then I haven't slept much lately anyhow, with the business and all. But I did think a lot about you, Ginger."

"Why, Duke?"

"Maggie was not only your sister but your best friend."

"I know, but I think I came to terms that Maggie was gone a while ago. At least the Maggie who we knew, the loving and caring Maggie. I came to realize it when she wanted to know who she was. When she said, "Who am I, and What am I doing here?" I realized she was gone that her spirit, her passion, was gone.

She didn't know anymore. She didn't recognize us. She didn't even remember the house she was born and raised in. She lost her identity and purpose, her reason for living - I guess. And that's when I think she was gone. Oh! I don't know. It's all a blur."

Sorry, Duke, not in the mood for the eggs, but I will finish the bacon."

"That's OK, Ginger. Maxx, how are those pancakes?"

"Pancakes are good, thanks.

I think the same thing, Ginger. Maggie was gone before she died. And you know what, I am so happy that you were there for her. You were there for her through the thick and the thin of it. You never left her side and always held her hand. Whether her personality was there or not, whether she consciously knew who she was, or what her purpose was, her soul and spirit knew that you were there for her to the last moment."

"We love you, Ginger, and we love Maggie too," whispered Duke.

"Let's say we leave in fifteen minutes for Maggie's service?" offered Maxx.

"Give me 20 guys. I need twenty minutes, uttered Duke."

At the same moment, both Ginger and Maxx said, "No problem!"

But Ginger blurted out, "You owe me a Coke."

Just then, all three gave a hearty and much-needed laugh.

"Okie Dokie," agreed Duke."

"Oh, Duke, I forgot to mention. I won't be able to meet with you to talk about the seven strategies next weekend. Sorry, we kind of lost touch and forgot over the past few days. We would have to discuss it in about two or three weeks. I was asked by "Sunshine Dementia" to return to their headquarters in Florida for some more consulting. It seems like they had some executive management changes, and the new administration wants to get certified as a Dementia Friendly Facility™ and are proposing I head off the effort. They have a problem where two higher-level leaders who did not buy into the new vision and left. They were both old enough to retire or something like that. It will take a couple of weeks. Is that good with you?"

"That's OK, Maxx. Give me a call when you are ready to sit and discuss the formula in detail."

"Duke, I will give you a portfolio, explaining the seven strategies in detail. Read it two or three times. Take notes. And we will discuss how to start implementing the program."

"So you know, I have officially taken on consulting in transforming home care, hospice, and assisted living companies into dementia focused organizations. It's a niche that I am passionate about. The more companies I can help in serving the patients and families, the better. Oh! I won't sell my services to anyone in your area. You have an exclusive - I promise.

I have some news about Wellspring Senior Care and the Dementia Friendly Facility™ system. But I am sworn to secrecy. I am working on a project with them, and I will let you know soon. I will say they are very passionate about serving those who serve others in the dementia healthcare field. 'Nuff said."

"Maxx, that all sounds great. I can tell that you are passionate about serving and want to serve others. Good luck, and I look forward to making your plan part of our vision strategy. When are you leaving?"

"Well, they wanted me today. But of course, I told them no. I will be leaving on the first flight out in the morning. I think it's somewhere around 7 a.m. out of JFK airport."

"OK, Maxx, well, I am ready. Ginger, let's go to church and say goodbye to Maggie."

PART TWO

SEVEN SIMPLE STRATEGIES FOR LEADING DEMENTIA CARE IN ASSISTED LIVING, HOSPICE, AND HOME CARE

MAXX'S ADVICE FOR DUKE

CHRISTOPHER SMITH   WHO AM I AND WHAT AM I DOING HERE?

Introduction

"Everyone has the potential to be a leader, to inspire others in their actions and their compassion towards others." – Christopher Smith.

Here are some quick and simple notes on leadership for managers, directors, team leaders, case managers, and those on the front line who aspire towards greatness in their field. Even though my experience is within the home care, hospice, and assisted living fields, the concepts are the same for all senior healthcare. Whether you are a director of a dining room at an assisted living center, a case manager for a hospice organization, a volunteer coordinator for a home health care organization, and everyone in between, these notes are for you.

No matter your position or role, either as a manager, supervisor, team leader, regional director, the lead aide, nursing case manager, or any other place in senior healthcare that has individuals working 'with' you under your guidance and support, I salute you and thank you. I encourage you to follow your passion, especially if you feel the desire to lead and inspire others.

My original intent was to tell a short story that would reflect some of the challenges in a dying dementia patient's healthcare field. And as I was writing, I was taking these notes on the side. After reviewing my notes, I then decided to add them to this book. I added an extensive appendix for you that offers additional information for follow-up reading and research.

Whether you have hundreds of people under you or one other person besides yourself, you influence others' lives, and by my definition, you are a leader. Therefore, the concepts you find here will apply to you.

They say that the tiniest little brush of air from a butterfly's wings can cause a change in an event around the world. In The Vocation of Man (1800), Johann Gottlieb Fichte says, "you could not remove a single grain of sand from its place without thereby changing something throughout all parts of the immeasurable whole." Assuming these statements are half-true, there can be exponential effects on the power, inspiration, and motivation, as small as you think it might be, not only among the individuals with whom you interact and have relationships but also with the people with whom they interact with and serve.

Whether you belong to a small business of only a few dozen employees, a franchise, or a national organization with thousands of healthcare workers, the concepts once applied will enhance and expand towards anyone who has a patient and their families at the core of their service.

As a senior healthcare and dementia care leader, you are sometimes alone facing similar challenges that a national or international organization leader faces every day. The difference is the larger organizational leader has many people within their organizations from which to gather support.

You, the nurse manager of that local hospice, the executive director of that assisted living facility, or the franchise owner of that home care are challenged daily on the tough decisions of putting out fires of compliance, supporting an aide in caring for a dying patient, or listening to a patient complain about the dining room food.

The daily questions, whether you know them or not, are: Which is more important? Which is the priority? And To whom? Which focus' would serve the vision best? Only you can answer that question, and even though the situations may be similar, each day has its own set of priorities forcing you to make difficult decisions.

You may base those decisions in large part based on how well you lead towards the organization's vision or how easily you are drawn towards the 'fire' called compliance. Similar to the way a moth is drawn towards the bright light of a flame.

Your attitude, the attitude of the leader, is essential to move forward; it is the first step. The wrong or poor attitude will not allow you to advance in a manner that would serve you, the organization, its employees, or the community. It just won't work. Oh, it may work for a short while, but failure is inevitable. Attitude is essential for success. You don't have to call it servant leadership. Call it what you like but, just don't get lost in the legalism of the definition.

The attitude of a leader in the senior and dementia healthcare field must be one of serving others. Think about it - why would anyone get involved in the healthcare field if they did not have a desire, an attitude, to serve others. Understand you have an internal desire that drives you to do what you do, do what you see possible, and care for others. Once you start feeding that drive, then you live your passion; it's an attitude, motivation, and inspiration in everything you do. Your mindset to lead and inspire others is the essential internal motivation that acts on your values and beliefs.

As you read through the leadership strategies and feel a fire burning, you may have some internal passion lighting up. Follow it, let it lead you to serve others and those with whom you work.

The following seven essential leadership qualities presented are not all-inclusive but represent some of what I believe are a few of the higher-level character traits that I sense are critical to the home-care, assisted living, and hospice organizations of the future. Although there are more, many more, you can only focus on one or two at a time. As you progress and move forward, other leadership qualities inherent in you will emerge, and they will emerge naturally.

Important note: When an individual leader, and this is for all levels of leadership and management, focus on these seven strategies, as a bonus, they will improve on other areas of their personal life. Your relationships will improve. As your light grows, you will see the light in others increase as well. You will notice possibilities and opportunities and see the good in others. A leader is a personality trait as well as an organizational role. It is the person, not necessarily a title or the position. And that is where we start - the leader, the individual servant leader.

My suggestion would be to read and understand all of the qualities, maybe read it more than twice. Since you want these aspects to be a part of your daily rituals, a one-time reading will not suffice. Afterwards go back and focus on one aspect first, making it a priority, then two weeks later, add the second, with a focus on the second while still incorporating the first. Then add one to two strategies after that one, and so on. Watch how fast and efficiently you absorb the concepts into your life, and each time they become easier to incorporate into your daily actions and behaviors. Watch how you change, and your employees change with you. Over time, you will see the trickle-down effect of the organization changing.

You will need to put time into change. If you truly have the passion and the fire to change, you will. That's why I put chameleon as number two before vision. If you have the passion, but you don't accept that you must change, accepting change in yourself first, then conveying the vision with passion will not work.

The book is not finished in the last chapter. I have added an appendix with important information for you. I have listed only a few books that I would strongly recommend you read to supplement our discussion and added mini leadership questionnaire to help you understand yourself. I have also included an introduction to the Certified Dementia Care Leader program and the Dementia Friendly Facility™ assessment and certification system. And then there is 'some of the stories behind the story.'

If you have a passion for serving others in senior care, especially the dementia care field, this book and the supporting material will support you in the knowledge, inspiration, and support you may need.

God Bless You In Your Journey,

Christopher Smith

Chapter One

Attitude And The Servant Leader

> *"A noble leader answers not to the trumpet calls of self-promotion, but to the hushed whispers of necessity."* — Mollie Marti.

> *"Attitude is a little thing that makes a big difference."* - Winston Churchill.

The 'attitude of the leader' for this book's terms herein assumes servant leader - which is not a role, a title, or position. There are no rules and regulations, no job description or requirements. A servant leader is one whose attitude is to serve others first (period). Not second, third, not after but first. They understand that the bottom line, the profits are not the only goal. To achieve profits, they must first achieve a positive relationship with the employees. In turn, they will return a profit from treating the customer with dignity, respect, and admiration. Relationships first.

As for me, I frequently state the leader '"must love their employees." Of course, this is not physical love but brotherly love, a respect that is higher than just a professional courtesy, but one that knows we are connected and gifted to serve with compassion and caring for a clearly focused group of individuals.

In the senior and dementia care field, whether it be home health care, hospice, assisted living, nursing homes, rehabilitation facilities, adult day care, or even a hospital setting; if we don't love the employees, if we cannot treat them with the utmost respect and dignity, then we are in the wrong business.

The qualities that we want to see in our front-line staff are the qualities we should first visit within ourselves and our leadership. Self-serving, power-hungry, controlling, manipulative, micro-management of employees focusing on profits, compliance, and insurance regulations will result in unsatisfied or apathetic employees who minimally care for the patients and families.

Being compliant and profit-driven is not empowering, nor does it allow for regular, ongoing, and consistent growth in the long term.

When you realize that higher profits come directly from employee efforts, you have tapped into a higher calling. Once you recognize where the profits are made, then your calling is to serve others. When you lay out the organization's vision and goals to your next level leaders and managers and the rest of the organization, everyone should know where they are going and what they are doing. Most importantly, they should know who they are and their worth within your organization.

Servant leaders walk the talk, know their subordinates, and shake hands, thanking them daily and regularly. They don't get pulled into the downward spiral of predominately relying on tech-no-speak communication to people through email, Facebook, LinkedIn, Twitter, or any other source other than face-to-face conversations.

Would you allow your front-line staff to care for the customer using technology instead of face-to-face? Although this book was several years in the making, I took pen to paper. I wrote this book at the start of the Covid-19 pandemic, where many healthcare workers, including myself, were restricted from contacting their regular patients. Televisits became the norm, communicating via phone or a technology-based service. The clinical side was done over the phone. After many conversations with the clinical team, there was frustration in not getting the full picture. The clinical staff could not get heart rates, take pulses, blood pressure readings, and more importantly, they could not see the facial expressions and tone of the patients. The heart of the matter, not the beating heart but the heart that ties us all together, was missing.

I was asked to make phone calls to front line employees: mostly aides and caregivers. After calling several dozen employees, the most common response was that the front line did not hear from management, and they felt that no one cared about them. Even though I was not management, they were relieved. I heard it in their voice, in their tone - there was a sigh of relief. After those many conversations, it became real. The heart of the matter was important for the clinicians and front line caregivers as it was for the patient.

This same concept holds for you as the manager, director, or team leader. You cannot fully understand and appreciate those who work with you or are subordinate to your role without face-to-face contact. This is an attitude - without the attitude of passion in building relationships with your employees and co-workers, you will lack the desire to serve the patient and families. One does not work well without 'the others'.

Your conversations with your staff need to reflect and mirror how you would like to see them behave with your patients and families. People want to know that leadership cares whether they are called leaders or managers or directors; it doesn't matter. It's less about what you say and more about what you do, both behind the scenes and in full view.

As a leader, there are two big concepts that we have touched on but will return to in the following notes. The first is the vision and the strategic plan. This is where the strategic skills of the leader come into play. If you don't have a vision, you do not have a big picture to communicate to the employees and the customer. Every department and every project can create a vision as long as it ties into the organization's overarching vision. The next part of the strategic plan are the goals and action plan. These are always a work in process and should be examined and updated regularly. The vision, however, does not change. It becomes achievable through the goals and actions. This is called strategic leadership, which is an element of the leader.

The servant leader, the 'whole' leader of any department, project, region, or organization, gets down and dirty and discovers those aspects needed by the front-line employees to do their jobs and be successful. When the servant leader is on the vision journey towards his employees, the leader is always asking, "What can I do for you?". The emphasis here is on 'always'. This is a lifelong journey as long as the leader is in a leadership position.

Ken Blanchard stated this well,

"In a traditional organization, all the energy in the organization moves up the hierarchical pyramid as people try to be responsive to their bosses instead of focusing their energy on meeting the needs of their customers. Bureaucracy rules and policies and procedures carry the day.

This creates unprepared and uncommitted customer contact people trying to protect themselves, leaving customers uncared for at the bottom of the hierarchy. This scenario doesn't do much to move the organization in the desired direction toward accomplishing a clear vision. Servant leaders, on the other hand, feel their role is to help people achieve their goals. In order to help people succeed in that manner, the traditional hierarchical pyramid is theoretically turned upside down so that the front-line people, who are closest to the customers, are at the top. Now the front-line people are responsible--able to respond--to the needs of the customers. In this scenario, leaders serve and are responsive to their people's needs, training and developing them to accomplish established goals and live according to the vision.

Servant leadership is not soft management; it is management that gets not only great results but also generates great human satisfaction."

Servant leadership is a place that allows you to let your light shine on your employees so they can see clearly. This will enable them to realize the success they possess within themselves in serving the patients and families.

Leaders with the right attitude:

Ask questions:

1. What can I do for you today?
2. How are you holding up?
3. What are you working on today?
4. How are you feeling today?
5. Are pro-active listeners listening? Not to come up with a solution or answer to their problems, but with a heart of compassion.

People want to know you care, and they are an essential part of the organization.
People want to know they matter.

> "Action springs not from thought, but a readiness for responsibility." —
> *Dietrich Bonhoeffer.*

Chapter Two

The Three Spheres of Focus

- **Leadership**
- **Marketing**
- **Training and Development**

"Show Us, Don't Tell Us." - Miles Anthony Smith.

Leadership - The First Sphere

> *"Are we going to order our inner worlds, our hearts, so that they will radiate influence into the outer world? Or will we neglect our private worlds and, thus, permit the outer influences to shape us? This is a choice we must make every day of our lives."* — Gordon MacDonald, Ordering Your Private World.

We have already discussed leadership in the previous section, and we will discuss aspects of leadership with some recommendations in the seven strategies coming up in the next section. Leadership is so significant and covers so much that it has an enormous impact on people and the organization that the conversations overlap in several areas. In this chapter, I would like to focus on a more general overview of leadership in hospice, home-care, and assisted living. Keep in mind that these are not necessarily the absolute top three, but they are the ones that I feel are important.

In this area of focus, leadership is, without a doubt, the individuals' attitude on top of the organization's hierarchy. My premise is that it is as much an attitude of those in other positions: the managers, directors, project leaders, and team leaders. Those individuals like dining room directors, environmental directors and managers, regional managers, nursing aide team leaders, maintenance and facility managers, and others responsible for organizing, maintaining, and supporting staff that in some way care for patients and families. If they decide to be a servant leader, all of these roles decide to make it a lifestyle. It would be inherent and built into everything they say and do. It's concepts, behaviors, and attitudes carry onward, sideways, upward, and downward into all areas of the organization and their lives. It encompasses the strategic plan, the vision, mission, values, targets, goals, actions, and behaviors of every department, team, and employee. It has far-reaching benefits and can change lives.

Like the breadth of the wings of a butterfly, servant leaders have the potential to change lives.

As you move through the rest of this plan, keep in mind the people about which the words speak.

Some of the characteristics of those employees that are led by the compliance-driven, bottom-line mentality. These employees:

- struggle with aligning values
- have trouble identifying important issues
- scheduling priorities
- work more than they need to
- are not as productive as they could be
- are usually overwhelmed and frustrated

They feel the need to focus on appearing busy as a measure of success and are usually looking to impress others. They set goals and targets based on their plan without thinking of others, and this is generally for the short term. They are always looking to do more and better for themselves as opposed to bettering others. They tend to be controlling, manipulative, micro-managing, and highly competitive against others instead of themselves. They hire people like themselves, who are puppets.

The 'puppet brigade' anticipates the managers' wishes and desires in advance, hoping to get an upper-hand on the next step. They listen and react without questioning, in fear of retaliation, demotion, or being fired.

These 'driven' people have trouble with anger and emotions, even though they may control their behaviors to a degree. They still harbor internal frustrations and anxieties released at the wrong time and on the wrong people, whether at home or work.

These are people who are driven, a concept explained by Gordon McDonald in his book, *Ordering Your Private World*. Gordon describes the difference between someone who is called and someone who is driven. A called leader realizes that there is a higher person and a higher level of purpose for which he or she must serve. A called leader realizes that everything is on loan, nothing is theirs, and it is their job to make the best of all resources - especially people.

Leaders at the front line in senior and dementia healthcare must realize that the people who work for us, the organization, and ultimately the patient and families - each and everyone - are on loan to us, and we are on loan to them. And since they are on loan, we should treat them as if we need to return them better than they came to us.

Look at your employees as a resource. You are paying them to work. Wouldn't it be more beneficial to think of them as a resource to empower as opposed to someone you should expect a return on for your payment? If you are looking for a return, you will always look for more - seeking higher profits - and getting back the same, if not less.

But if you look at them as an investment, you will treat them with a higher level of purpose. When you buy a car, it depreciates when you drive it out of the lot - and continues to depreciate. Seldom can a car offer a positive return on your investment? In actuality, a car is not an investment but a liability. Yet, many individuals will use that car as a status symbol, bring it to the car wash and make sure it's nice and shiny - spending (not investing) more money.

Yet, the employee, a resource that can increase your profits, may not be treated by many managers as well as they treat their cars.

Driven people make their cars shiny.

'Called leaders' shine the light on their employees.

Marketing - The Second Sphere

To Be a Great Marketer, You Have to Be a Great Leader First - Jon Miller

This area of focus is the other one that is ongoing and must be toiled every day. It needs to be tended to, worked on, analyzed, and mastered. You need to be creative in all areas except one. Your heart must be steadfast and needs to be true to the vision and the care of the patient, caregiver, and families of the future.

Isn't that what marketing is? Serving the customers of the future. Yes, marketing is serving. As a leader, you are educating, informing, and inspiring. And an important note, all levels of management who see themselves as leaders are marketing. Marketing is inspiring, and if you inspire others, you are a leader.

Together let's take a look at an example:

Dining room - anyone can place a fork and knife in the right order, yet it's a learned skill. Cooking a meal is also a skill that is learned. Now watch those people who have a passion for their work in the dining room. It's easy to see them - they have smiles on their face, a spring in their step, and move with grace. Ask them why they are passionate about their work. Guarantee that they will say something that has to do with relationships, probably the 'serving' of others. I would also venture to guess that these individuals who 'serve' have a light on them in many conversations among the residents and patients.

As you are reading this, I am sure you can think of someone in your organization that has a 'spring in their step'. It could be an aide, maintenance worker, nurse, or gardener. These individuals are a delight to others, even in the smallest way. And they are known and can be seen in action by others. Isn't that what marketing is - getting others to see and talk about your business? It's about attitude first and foremost. It's about passion and being called.

Leaders are called to be marketers, maybe not as a skill set, but as an attitude in how they inspire others with the 'spring in their step' and 'grace in their movement.' They walk-the-talk as if there is always a light shining on them.

Educating is also part of marketing, especially in the dementia field. Not only for the dementia patients and families but also for those employees working within the technical aspects of home-care, assisted living, and hospice. Education, which includes training, coaching, and consulting, is vital to each individual and the organization as a whole.

As a marketer, you may already know that your future client is scared, frustrated, and anxious. Your job is to ease their fears and help them to understand what is going on right now and how you can help them in the future. Your job is to explain, without actually saying so, how your expertise in the field of healthcare and dementia sets you apart from everyone else.

Caution, do not fix them - dementia can't be fixed. Dementia has a life, and it's own journey. Once patients and families decide to choose you as their professional support system, then you become part of their family on the journey with them. And that's what they want, trust and hand-holding. They want to know that they will not be betrayed and forgotten. When speaking of dementia patients and families, the operative phrase is that they don't want to be 'forgotten.' Even though they may not say that or imply it, being forgotten is just as frightening as forgetting.

Let me repeat that being forgotten is just as frightening as forgetting.

Marketing dementia services either with you as the dementia expert, someone that leads this project, an outside consultant, or a director of your organization, you are the face of your organizations' professionalism and specialization. Once the patient and family have signed on, many marketing individuals fall away and are no longer seen. I have seen this in every organization I have worked for.

I have heard this many times, not as a complaint but a comment when referring to the marketing specialist: "I was hoping to see them again." Or "Are they still with your company? I have not heard from them." Since many marketers come on strong and are persistent at the beginning of their relationship with the patient and family, being, overly friendly, and seemingly concerned, they build a strong connection in eyes of that patient and family.

A dementia specialist who should be part of the marketing team should not fall off as soon as the family signs on the bottom line. They are part of the team, in regular and ongoing contact. Don't make the mistake of the 'community representatives' falling off the grid. They are part of the family and should remain with them on their journey.

Marketing representatives should maintain regular and ongoing relationships with the teams. Since all organization members are marketing, why not let them be in regular contact with those at the front line. Those who have regular, daily contact with the patients and families. Why shouldn't the nurse's aides have an ongoing friendly relationship with the marketing people?

I know that patients and families have been referred by the nurse aides of those organizations with which I have had associations.

Yet, these front line staff were not always comfortable with whom to turn. Imagine if they were given an individual with whom they have had contact, with whom they have an ongoing relationship. Imagine if those simple and easy referrals doubled. As a servant leader, that is, serving the front-line staff and the patients and families.

A 'stop doing' item: Stop sending food to doctors' offices. The 'we will buy you lunch if you let us tell you about our business' is a bribe - stop it! It's needy and does not come off very well. You don't look like the 'experts' or 'specialist' in the field. Just another home-care, hospice, or assisted living looking for business. It's tacky - stop it! I have seen this backfire a few times. 'Nuff said.

As the dementia expert in your organization, you must educate, inform, inspire.

Question?

What percentage of your patient base is diagnosed with dementia as a primary or secondary disease? Is that percentage at least equal to or more than the dementia training of your marketing team?

You can't serve that which you do not know, appreciate, and understand.

Every week, at a minimum, your key marketing players should be teaching or speaking somewhere. In between, they should be coaching and mentoring. With whom do your key players present every week? They will present to anyone who may become a patient or have a family member become a patient within three to seven years.

Some ideas:

- Hook up with churches to set up a training program to teach volunteers visitation.
- Book annual presentations at Rotary clubs, Lions clubs, and senior centers. There is enough there to book yourself for every week of the year.
- Schools, community centers, adult education centers - teach, speak, train, coach.
- Present and teach at local hospitals, assisted living facilities and nursing homes
- Partner with like organizations to lead and hold one-day fairs, or seminars
- Become the 'top of mind,' 'go-to' organization as 'experts' in dementia care.
- Besides training every single one of your employees (more on that later), offer to do an annual training at each assisted living, nursing home, or hospital, free. Yes, free and make it a certification class with follow-up CEU in-services and schedule it a year in advance. Before you know it, you are speaking or training somewhere every week.

As a consultant to home-care, hospice, and assisted living organizations, this is the primary way that I see you becoming the 'experts.' Using the Kaizen philosophy (more in that chapter later), you can own the market. Whenever someone thinks of dementia, home-care, assisted living, or hospice, they will think of you.

Like 'Band-Aids' and 'Q-tips'. If you need to cover a cut, you get a 'Band-Aid' or clean your ears or remove makeup, you grab a "Q-tip". When they speak of dementia, they should think of you.

Don'ts:

Don't stop learning - there is so much information out there on dementia that you can super niche yourself as the expert in the field of dementia - find it, learn it - do it!

Don't stop speaking - every week, present something somewhere. Always have your calendar booked and always make it available for the public to view.

Don't buy food. Well, it's OK to buy food when you are presenting but not 'just' food.

Some time ago, a home-care company wanted to get noticed by a local assisted living center. They bought lunch or fun snacks for the employees every week, and they had the deli that made lunch and snacks deliver the food. The home-care company never came when the food arrived. But guess who did? Me! And every time they brought food, I showed up - creating relationships and bonded. I helped serve or assist if I could. Who do you think the people remembered? Right - the relationship! After several months, the assisted living gave the home-care a try with a contract. Two months later, they were kicked out because they did the absolute minimum and had little relationships with the staff and patients.

Don't stop creating relationships - most of the time, all it takes is listening and caring.

Don't stop listening - sorry if this is rude but 'shut up and listen'!

Some individuals should be listening and learning from those they serve instead of speaking. Individuals who talk too much begin to control the communication fueling their plan instead of focusing on those they should be serving. They never get to the heart of the matter. These people have their schedule and mask it well to make it look like they care. Listen with empathy. If you are reading this far, then I would guess that you are seeking to improve yourself in this endeavor. These people tend to be 'lone wolves' working in 'silos.'

Be attentive, attaining, and acting.

- Attentive and listening with empathy
- Attaining information and learning with the intent to serve without an agenda
- Acting with intent to serve and care

The emphasis here is on no list - if you have no plan, you should have little to say.

Don't stop serving. Keep serving. What can you do for others? Don't make this a mantra - you must, I will repeat, you must make this a matter of the heart, not the mind. Remember, you are not in a sales job. As a dementia care specialist, your experience and love for those you serve are already essential for you; just make sure this part of your role is in getting the word out so others can learn, understand, and appreciate it. And when the time is right, when they need dementia support, they will think of you.

Training and Development - The Third Sphere

> *"Leadership and learning are indispensable to each other."*
> John F. Kennedy.

The individual in the leadership position who is poised to present this program should have the training and advanced education as a dementia care leader, teacher, trainer, consultant, or coach. Additional certifications are available that can be used to enhance and complement the training of employees and the community. As with strengths and gifts, the individual's education and certifications should show a propensity towards leadership, management, and dementia care.

To be clear, the focus as it pertains to this book is on leadership, not on the skills on specific caring details at the front line. Those are specific skills focused on the details in the personal care of the individual's physical needs.

More importantly, there is a growing field of knowledge in dementia. There will always be continuing and advancing pieces of knowledge with various ways of presenting that knowledge. It's a growing field, not necessarily by design but by demand. The 'silver tsunami' is approaching. It is the devastation of an oncoming 'dementia wave' that will affect most lives soon.

Face-to-Face first

Training and development of employees in understanding dementia should entail a basic training program for every employee. Yes, everyone - from maintenance to the c-suite and everyone in-between. There may be different training levels, depending on the level, intensity, and regularity of contact with dementia patients, yet everyone should have training. If they are employed by an organization that cares for those patients and families, they must be trained.

All employees should have face-to-face contact with the trainer and coach, whether that trainer and coach is the leader or director or is from an outside consulting service. In other words, the initial training for any individual should include live interactive training with individuals seeking the same goal of the program. Interactive live training allows for practical and useful skills to be learned. An excellent interactive program will keep participants engaged and learning at a higher level. When offered regularly and consistently, I feel that online training can help the learning effectiveness of those at the front line in senior care and caring for our friends with dementia.

I completed this book during the Covid-19 pandemic. On-line training has skyrocketed. With that, on-line training will develop, and I see the future of on-line training as becoming a practical and useful tool. A good, well-trained facilitator and coach can effectively engage participants and create a learning-intensive and effective environment. On-line training will not replace face-to-face engaging workshops, especially personalized 'learning', but they are an excellent second-best option.

Finding a program that is engaging is challenging. I have been a participant in certifications that were live. The facilitator read from the power points for two days, and it was the most troublesome certification I have ever attended. Then I attended other workshops, specifically in leadership training. There was intensive, interactive, high-contact learning, almost non-stop for two and a half days, twelve hours each day. It appeared like it was only a few hours. To this day, I reap the rewards of that learning and the desire to facilitate my workshops similarly. High-performance workshops lead by a highly interactive facilitator will be a reward for you and your employees that can be immeasurable.

All staff training should be ongoing and regular with a routine supportive program that will advance and support its needs. The best programs are those personalized for the individual, designed around the facility or organizational needs. The front-line staff training should include a comprehensive basic program with a follow up continuing education program specific to your organization (see below).

Appreciation Certification

Those individuals who are not in daily direct contact with the patients and families should have an in-house appreciation certification program that will be a broad stroke of the comprehensive program that the front-line receives. The support staff should have an understanding of dementia and care, as well as a sense of what the front-line staff is learning.

Additionally, as a part of the appreciation certification, all support staff should 'shadow' a front-line staff at a minimum of once a year for a full day as necessary for the second part of the in-house certification. This is not cross-training but appreciation training. I have seen this as a big part of our system of learning, and it is indispensable. It creates awareness, understanding and deepens the relationship of the employees.

As the leader of this program, watch how the appreciation learning changes the support staff's behaviors - especially after shadowing. You will see a higher level of compassion and empathy towards the patients, families, and front-line staff. Conduct a feedback meeting for fun and enjoyment and see what happens.

Continuing education - should be ongoing and regular with options for face-to-face seminars, workshops, and online programs. Additionally, having staff teach other staff should be a goal as the program progresses. You will find that the coaching and teaching potential will arise out of a few employees. These employee's enthusiasm will make a continuing education as part of your dementia program an enjoyable success.

Corporate certification - a corporate certification program creates:

- **Brand awareness** with your employees because every employee is a salesperson, and it is essential that they get to know your company well.
- **There should be a strong bond** and allegiance not only with the organization but with other employees.

If structured well, an ongoing and consistent training and development program:

- **Gives the employees options** to improve their growth and development that would complement their service in your organization, improving their relationships with the families and patients.
- Offers your organization a **strong voice and a competitive edge** - confidently and honestly calling the organization the 'expert' and 'specialist' in the field of dementia care.
- Be aware that there are home care and hospice organizations that call themselves experts, but when you review their websites or know who they are - they are bending the truth.
- **Builds credibility** within the community and your employees. It shows that you do what you say - that you walk the talk.
- **Reduces turnover** - a company that will invest in the training and development of their employees is a company that cares for its employees as well as the people they serve. People don't leave companies that care for them. Employees leave companies because the management does not care for them, where they have no support, no appreciation, no recognition, and no purpose.

Another word about leadership.

Leadership must have 110% buy-in from all levels to implement this program. If you are a director or manager, you may need that approval to move forward. But I believe you need more. You may need to have realized the passion for the potential of the program. To be the experts and specialists in this field, the leaders must all backup and support the program. There will be individuals from leadership, support staff, and front-line staff who will push back and say they don't need support or training. They will say they have been working in the field long enough to know. The only exception is those who have achieved certification themselves - and those individuals, you will see, will become the rising stars in the program and have a desire to learn more.

When you have 'naysayers,' you need confidence to state that the program is a mandate, approved and supported by upper management and leadership. That's why you need the support of the top leaders of the organization. Without the support of top leadership, you will not have the confidence to lead the program with honesty and integrity. It is worth the effort to get the support you need to succeed.

When the front line and support classes are rolled out, have an essential member of the top leadership who already have 'buy-in,' lead by example, and attend the workshops with the employees - strategically placed so that the employees are aware that the top leaders are serious about the new vision.

Recognition *versus* ***Appreciation****:*
Employees need both - know the difference.

Recognition is an acknowledgment of their job or duties. Your recognition validates their work.

Appreciation is an act of showing gratitude to a person and who they are as an individual.

Recognition is concrete, tangible, and of the mind,
whereas appreciation is abstract and of the heart.
Recognition is temporary; appreciation runs deep and lasts longer.

Chapter Three

Seven Simple Strategies of Dementia Care Leadership

"Only a life lived in the service to others is worth living." - Albert Einstein.

- Passion
- Chameleon
- Vision
- Kaizen
- Effective
- Empowering
- Tribe, Teams, Silos, and Wolves

Passion – The First Strategy

> *"Nothing is as important as passion. No matter what you want to do with your life, be passionate." - Jon Bon Jovi.*

The first strategy is passion and being passionate about the needs of the patient and family and passionate about how effective you are in caring for them, making the aspects of what you do better, faster, and more effective and not efficient. Being efficient, a management function often seen in senior healthcare compliance and insurance regulations, could be a killer of effectiveness (*and compassion*).

Passion is intimate; it's a burning desire; it's deep and meaningful. Although it can't be seen, except in the individual's behaviors and energy, it surely can be felt. It's the energy that can be shared and multiplied and, if nurtured regularly, can seldom burn out.

When I was in my early thirties, I was struggling as a computer network consultant. I was getting paid very well and enjoyed my work. However, I was unhappy. When an organization hired me, they went into detail about my experience, education, and training. Several individuals usually interviewed me until I was awarded the contract. In many cases, not all, I would be asked for my recommendation, and based on that recommendation, I would be asked to head the project.

One of my biggest joys, then and now, is to put a project together. I love to see progress with a group of people who started with a thought and developed that thought into an achievable goal and then to its completion. I feel charged and energetic when I see progress. I lived for the journey and was always looking for the next big project in the middle of the current project.

My frustration came when the recommendations that developed into projects repeatedly led to a downturn when someone was trying to circumvent or undermine the project. In most cases, that particular project would fail or at least run into so many complications that it went over budget.

During that time, I had a love and desire for fitness and health on the personal side of my life. It was a significant part of my lifestyle. I studied and was certified as a personal trainer with several organizations just for the fun of it. Two of them were the American College of Sports Medicine and the National Strength and Condition Association. After about two years, I successfully achieved over a dozen certifications in health, fitness, strength conditioning, and lifestyle management.

And for the fun of it, again, I started a health and fitness company where I was a vendor in health fairs measuring people's body composition and making fitness recommendations. It was fun and enjoyable. That turned into working as a personal trainer and then manager of a fitness facility. I loved the fitness business so much that I quit my computer consulting work and built and created a 25,000 square foot, two-floor, multi-faceted fitness facility.

The high energy, the challenge, and the desire to work with others, the commitment to my goals while helping others achieve their fitness goals were exhilarating. And I did not realize it at the time, but I was able to charge and stir positive energy in a contagious way. For me, passion comes from the strong desire to give away energy and help others live that energy in a way that works for them - transforming my energy and passion into their energy and passion.

And there is something else I found out about passion. Passion and love are two charges of energy. And when you have passion and love for your employees, that passion and love will be absorbed and transformed in a way that will serve the patients and families.

The Law of Thermodynamics states that energy is always conserved. It cannot be created or destroyed. In essence, energy can be converted from one form into another. In healthcare leadership, the energy you receive is recycled and used by your team members and then converted again to serve their team members and, finally, the patient. Hey, it's a law, so it must be correct. And in my experience, it works.

Passionate servant healthcare leaders know that employees come first and are most important. They also understand that the customer, the patient, and the family are the priority. Remember, employees are the most important; patients and families are the priority. The passion you have for your employee is the fuel that burns the fire of passion for the patients and families.

Suppose you make your customers the most critical aspect of your business and give them the highest priority. In that case, your fuel will die out quickly, and you will have nothing to motivate, inspire, and empower your employees. That's why you have your employees as the most important, and your patients are the priority.

Stated another way, passion for the employees fuels the passion for the patients and families. When a goldsmith purifies gold, do they put the priority on the gold or the fire? The priority is on the 'fire.' The goldsmith needs the fire - without the fire, the gold will not purify even though it is more important than the fire.

So without the customer, the priority - the employees cannot do their work. This is not to say that the customer is not important or that their needs cannot become a priority. When we make these distinctions, it will drive our behaviors and our answers in a direction that will allow us to serve the patient and the employees best. Both are satisfied; both are served to create a highly effective, high-performance system.

Passion is equally essential when casting the vision. In today's technology world, if you have a cell phone or smartphone and want to see an image in a larger setting, you can cast it onto a television or screen. Now instead of viewing the image or video by yourself, you are viewing it with others. That's called sharing.

Casting your vision with the passion embodied deep in your heart and soul is sharing your dreams, desires, goals, and mission with others. You get the opportunity to show others what you see by sharing with them the image of the vision that you see and feel. It is this drive that you have about your vision that will inspire and motivate others.

Qualities of a Passionate leader

Not all leaders excel in the same qualities. Here are a few of the top qualities of a passionate leader:

Optimist - The quality of being an optimist is the ability to envision a brighter future. They do not wallow in the mire of the past. They see issues and problems as challenges.

Tip: Words are powerful and carry intense meaning. Change your vocabulary by using the word 'challenge' instead of 'problem.' Problems appear insurmountable and stifle productivity.

> *But if you have a 'challenge,' you automatically and subconsciously begin to think about overcoming that 'challenge.'*

Focus – Passionate leaders work and focus towards a goal overcoming and anticipating challenges. Their energy comes from the laser focus of their vision and goals.

Dedication – Dedicated leaders believe in themselves, the vision, the organization, and their people. They invite challenge and don't circumvent them unless it's to accomplish a necessary goal.

Eagerness – Passionate leaders are always ready, willing, and able to learn from successes and failures, not only from themselves but also from others. They see failure as a learning experience and the war-wounds of a tried-and-true leader. They invite opportunities to learn from experience as well as increasing knowledge or skills from education.

Resonant - a term made famous by Daniel Goleman. Passionate leaders realize that their behaviors and actions impact others to guide and help others. Resonant leaders go forth - first. They practice what they preach and walk the talk.

Drive – passionate leaders produce the momentum that yields results. They acquire the necessary resources to do what needs to be done to fulfill the mission. This is especially true when gaining a 110% buy-in from leadership and the employees.

Perseverance – I have a coffee cup from which I drink for over 20 years. It reads, "Never, Never Give Up." Interestingly when I read that cup, I add another 'never.' Giving up means that you don't have the passion, the desire, the motivation - that you have lost sight of the vision. However, a persevering leader will not give up when faced with failure. They always have a vision in mind. Passionate leaders do all they can to accomplish the goal and the result. A passionate leader can slow down and take a break, but they do not give up.

Never, Never, Never Give Up!

Enthusiasm - a passionate leader has deep within themselves the ability to make visions come alive. They breathe life into the vision through the energy in their actions, behaviors, and relationships. Enthusiasm is infectious, breeds motivation, and adds to the inspiration of the vision.

Chameleon – The Second Strategy

"You must be the change you want to see in the world." - Mahatma Gandhi.

After several years working as a computer consultant, it was challenging to go to work. There was nothing that fired me up. I started noticing that my focus was not where it should be. At that time, I started to realize and understand my strengths and gifts and began to write life goals. And not soon after that, I started to change. My attitude adjusted; my perception of my work changed. There was hope and significance in my life.

I started to become aware of challenging opportunities, sought out mentors, looked for advice, and learned what I could in the business of fitness. I changed my outlook, and my environment changed, as well. Or I should say, I changed in my environment - but it seemed like my surroundings, the people and the places changed. Yet, they did not. I changed my focus, noticed my surroundings, discovered what was working and not working, and adjusted my vision, goals, action plan, and, ultimately, my relationships.

Chameleons change as well. If you ever watch a chameleon, you will see that they can change colors in 20 seconds. I was not so fast - it took me some time, but hey, the thought that started the process may have taken 20 seconds.

Chameleons (and leaders) adjust the way they communicate with the world around them. They are acutely sensitive to their surroundings. They adapt and conform, creating a place where they create change in themselves.

Chameleon leaders do not expect their surroundings to change for them.

Leaders must do the same by acclimating themselves and fine-tune how they behave in changing circumstances. Like the chameleon, they must be acutely aware of where they are and of those around them. As healthcare leaders, we must understand and appreciate employee levels while we enjoy their company.

Yes - enjoy their company. Each employee has a different position; even in the same department, the skill sets, experiences, and personalities bring a different color to the rainbow of service provided to the patients. When a leader is genuinely behaving like a chameleon, the leader becomes the follower. At least in appreciation and learning of the department, team, or individual worker.

Chameleons use their tongue to capture prey as it's the primary function.

Leaders must be quick to adapt and change. Like a chameleon, leaders should not be using their tongue for any reason beyond it's intended function except to serve. They should be listening objectively yet empathetically, with wisdom and humility, and be quick to respond - if and when necessary. Listening as a leader with an empathetic ear places the other person in a position of importance and respect.

Chameleons can use each eye independently with an almost 360-degree view. It allows them to see a bigger picture. Leaders must be able to see the vision as a whole and as parts of the whole. They must see the vision from each employee's eyes, each team, and each department.

Leaders must also have a 360-degree view of the world around them. They must view each employee as holding a small piece of a thread that, when viewed from the leader's 30,000-foot perspective - encapsulates a carefully woven, beautifully crafted tapestry.

The leaders' attention should be directed towards how employees learn from each other, from their patients, and their families, even more importantly, how you can help them learn. Learning is not teaching. Leaders are likened to facilitators, to learn and focus on the individual, whereas teaching is focused on the content presented. When we seek to enable others to learn, we are focused on who they are, where they are, and how we can support their discovery of the lesson. This is how the leader adjusts his world to accommodate the world of the individual.

As a healthcare field leader with a focus on dementia patients, your focus is not organizational. However, your mindset should be. Think of your team or your department as an organization. What changes are taking place? To see this, you must step back and view your team from a leadership perspective - not getting caught in the management mode.

Management modes focus is on processes and procedures. It is more focused on the day-to-day tactics of the front-line administration. This mindset is focused on maintaining and controlling the current situation. Its focus is short term.

The leadership model is more future and vision focused. It looks at the way things were yesterday, today, and how they may be tomorrow. It plans the processes of tomorrow with the management function to start today. In dementia healthcare, change is imminent and will happen. The number of people getting dementia, the number of home-care, hospice, assisted living centers opening, the costs and charges in insurance, the methods of care, and the advances of medicine guarantee that there will be a change. So how are you preparing? What is your vision? How are you serving your employees and co-workers in the service of the vision for the patient?

What does your current day look like? Are you investing your time in what happened yesterday? Are you worrying about responding to every email? Are you leading meetings on putting out fires and how to put them out? Or are you focused on planning for tomorrow and projecting that plan to your employees? Are you listening when you ask your front-line staff how they can make things better, easier, and more effective? How can the organization help you, the front line, serve the patients and families better?

What you do in the future will depend on how well you listen to your employees – today! Are you listening?

You change and adapt by keeping your heart with the customer, your pulse on the market, your eyes and ears on your employees, and your mind on the finances and regulations. Your spirit must be in the heart of the vision.

Change is in your future, and adapting to the future of your organization is in large part in the:

- Research: the listening, the understanding, and appreciating
- Development: the innovation, the practice, the failures, and successes
- Training: the learning and re-learning

If you and your organization are not listening, not practicing, and not learning, you are not growing.

I want to add; there is an overlap in the seven strategies. Each strategy will overlap, complimenting, and adding to one or each other. But to make them part of what you do, we separate them, to distinguish and understand them. When we step back, we will see later that each of these strategies are colors in a tapestry in the rainbow that you will cast over your business. Whose light will shine onto your employees for the benefit of the patients and the families?

Leaders must walk the talk. The dementia care initiative leader must change themselves first, and they will change the world around you. You must change how you think so that the change within you can allow you to take new and innovative actions, creating new habits, removing old thoughts and patterns.

Qualities of the Chameleon Leader

Communication: The number one leadership skill is communication, and within that is listening and communicating to gain trust and inspire.

Influence and Inspiration - Embrace and encourage change as it benefits the individual team member. Seek out opportunities for encouragement and motivation.

Compassion and Empathy - To love your employees and team members, a leader must have a heart for them. They have a desire to understand and relate to them on their level without a personal agenda.

Strategic Thinker - You must know the vision and mission. Where the organization sees itself and how your team, your employees are going to get there. When you maintain that focus and stay the course, any waves and storms that come your way may take you off the path, and you will adjust quickly. The chameleon leader can adapt to the oncoming wave.

Confidence and Integrity - As a strategic thinker, the leader has the knowledge, the understanding, and the experience, which gives them the faith to stay the course in an oncoming wave.

Vision – The Third Strategy

> *"Shared Thinking is Shared Leadership"* - John Maxwell

One of the best and first things I did when I realized I would get into the fitness business was to create a plan with a vision. A super big, humongous dream that I knew would someday turn into reality. The biggest mistake I made was telling the wrong people about that dream. Wow! I was knocked down and out with every single person with whom I shared this dream. Well, I learned the hard way to be selective on who you choose to share your dreams with.

Anyhow, I made a huge long-term dream by making it real. How? I wrote down with pen and paper, every detail. Then I made a list of smaller steps that lead to that dream. As I progressed, the dream became a plan to a vision. I think that is when I knew that there was no stopping me because it made the vision so real. I had to be flexible as there were many roadblocks and speed bumps I had to overcome. But I didn't give up and moved forward. One small step at a time, until the butterfly breeze turned into a reality.

I wasn't going to include vision in this section because we talk about it in the three areas, but then I realized, well, we need it. The promotion of the vision is of crucial importance, and it is always a priority.

We have already talked about vision and casting the vision to the department or organization, so let's clarify this topic, including the departmental strategic plan. A strategic plan can be performed for a project or team; it's not only delegated to the whole organization. It does not have to be complicated nor time-consuming and can be enjoyable. At a minimum, the organization itself should have a vision, mission, and values statement. With a departmental or project vision, we bring your passion up a notch by creating a vision and strategic plan for your team.

For example: If you are a memory care unit director, you can bring your team(s) together to create an exclusive vision for your department that still ties in with the organization's vision. The same can be said for the dining room, housekeeping, and maintenance departments.

Whether your group is new or has been around for a while; whether your position is new, being created, or has also been around for a time - it needs a vision, a mission, and a values statement specific to the department or the initiative. It must tie into, reflect, and appreciate the grand vision of the organization.

Rarely have I seen a department in any organization have its own vision or strategic plan. Yet, each department has its own set of rules and regulations on how to do business, who and how they hire, and a description of their customer. They may not be written down nor clearly defined in perfect wording, but they are understood. So why shouldn't each section of the organization have its own strategic plan?

A couple or a few hours together with key people can easily work to create a vision, mission, and a few values to focus the players into a more cohesive and aligned mission.

As the team leader, you must always motivate, inspire - talk the vision and mission, and walk-the-talk. You must sleep it, drink it, eat it, and breathe it. The vision should be in the DNA of your blood.

Recall our story in part one, when Maggie had those two episodes where she repeated, "Who am I?" and "What am I doing here?" Those statements, which are familiar with someone with dementia, made me think how important it is that we, as individuals in an organization and team members, need to understand our identity and purpose. We all need to know who we are, why we are at the organization, and how that ties together. The vision is a big part of answering that question.

The answer to the questions, "Who am I?" and "What am I doing here?" lie deeper than your title and job requirements. It has a deeper personal meaning that intrinsically ties into the team as a whole, each team member, and then the recipients of your service - the patient and family.

Think about this: While doing your daily work, is it natural for you to think that the work you are doing is essential to your team and team members? Or do you solely focus on the patient?

If this is natural for you, then you probably think of these following phrases or questions to yourself, subconsciously without knowing that you do:

1. Which members of my team need to know this vital information?

2. This information will help my team or team member do a better job, not only for the team but also for the patient as well.

3. The team, the patient, and the family will benefit if I share it with...

Unfortunately, I have witnessed individuals who believed they were an integral part of a team yet withheld information that was later discovered as necessary for other team members to perform their job effectively but never received the support. After finding out that the information they had could have been useful to other team members, they would chant, "I did not know that would help you, or laugh it off and say, "oh, I didn't think of that!". This kind of thought process does not lend itself to thinking about the final recipient or the team's efforts. It lends itself to the preservation of the individual. We will talk more about this later when we discuss lone wolves and silos.

The best football and basketball players in history always know their team members, where they are located, how they operate, and how they perform in certain situations. Key players are still ready to pass the ball and let the other player score for the team's benefit. Those team players who always want to make a score without intrinsically thinking and considering their fellow team members can never become key players.

The strategic plan serves the team by focusing on each other and the patient and family. It helps us see the flowers within the weeds, pulling out the weeds, and tending to the garden.

Here's a quick test, do one step at a time without reading the next step.

Step 1: In the room you are in right now, look around for the color green and brown.

Don't read the next step until you have done this first step.

Step 2: Without looking around, in your mind, identify those things that are the color red.

Chances are you can't because you were focusing on the green when in reality, the purpose wasn't clear until I identified the real intent in the second step.

That's what a strategic plan does. It identifies the real intent of everything that you do - everything - every little thing. Once you identify the strategic plan, see the vision with absolute clarity, identify the mission, and know beyond a shadow of a doubt what you need to do, then the values you identified are necessary to carry out the mission.

The vision, mission, and values will help you see the thread that ties you and your team members together and how what you do, works together in harmony for the patient and family.

A violin is a beautiful instrument. When played, it's music can be soothing and comforting.

A harp, frequently used in the 11th hour of a dying patient, relaxes the soul.

A saxophone and trumpet can each cool your mojo and make you feel warm and relaxed at the same time.

Drums or bongos can play at a beat to your step.

Individually, these instruments make a sound that is unique and special. When orchestrated by a conductor, they collectively lead us to a pleasant and beautiful place. At the conductor's hands, the instruments are unified, where a tone and beat is maintained to achieve a single sound. Yet, that single sound can only be achieved by the single achievement of each musician.

(sidebar: the instruments - the tools, do not make the sound. It's the musician's talent and skills that create the sound in harmony with the instrument.)

The vision for the orchestra is the final masterpiece. When the conductor first formed the ensemble, the conductor introduced the vision. He identified the mission of the team and of each individual. They understand how their music and their mission ties into the vision. After daily leadership from the conductor, the musicians work together, and the masterpiece unfolds.

Within your dementia care team, you bring a unique set of skills and talents together. Adding your strengths and gifts, in harmony with your team members, you become woven together (not entangled) to create a beautiful tapestry that can be seen and appreciated by your team and the patients.

When you value others, you, the leader, will value their ideas.

John Maxwell, in his book '*Thinking for A Change*,' talks about sharing ideas and valuing the ideas of others. He states," *...believe that the ideas of other people have value. If you don't, your hands will be tied.*"

Qualities of a Vision Focused Leader:

Value in People: Vision focused leaders value each team member and their worth as an integral part of the vision.

Secure and Confident: Vision leaders are emotionally secure and confident in who they are and their roles as a leader.

High Importance: Vision focused leaders place higher importance on the team members, individually and collectively. In this way, the better our friends with dementia are served.

Proactive Listeners: Vision leaders can interact with the individual and listen without shutting them down. They hear and are always seeking clarity in understanding.

Relationship Builder: The team leader is centered on building relationships with the heart of a servant leader towards the vision of the organization, and if they have one, the vision and mission of the team.

Kaizen – The Fourth Strategy

"When eating an elephant, take one bite at a time." - Creighton Abrams.

Every day, well, almost every day, I do something that will make me better than the day before, whether it's reading a single page in a book, listening to a self-help audiobook, or writing a few pages in my journal. Walking, exercise, and fitness often help me maintain a positive mindset. Even dieting, and I mean not losing weight dieting - and I am so done with that - but the right diet - eating healthy.

In preparing to write this book, I first committed myself to work on it for at least 15 minutes every morning. I learned that morning was the best time for me. I am a morning person. I am awake before 5 am, do some kind of fitness for about an hour, plan my day, and then work on the plan. By 8:30 am, I have completed a considerable portion of writing, working on new business, and other projects. The significant aspect of doing this every day gives me momentum for the rest of the day. My mindset is in the right place, and my body is also in the right state. When challenges present themselves, they become easy to surmount or at least easier than if I was not prepared.

I look at my morning routine as the soft breeze that the wave of a butterfly offers to this world. It's noticeable only by me. Yet like the butterfly that stops fluttering its wings and perches on a branch, I feel that when I pause, I see my part in this world as a small part in a beautiful place with wonderful people.

This chapter is about making regular, ongoing, and consistent changes daily - the Kaizen mindset. To rephrase the opening quote from this chapter, if we take small, incremental bites every day, we will eat the elephant.

In the three spheres section of this book, I pointed to this philosophy in the marketing sphere. It is the small, ongoing, and incremental strategic placements of the marketing team's efforts that can benefit from this mindset.

Kaizen is a way of thinking that originated in the Japanese philosophy of lean manufacturing. It involves the whole organization in all stages of the process of the business. It's an understanding that small change eventually creates a considerable change over time for the customer's value.

For this discussion and this book, Kaizen is the leaders' ongoing, regular and consistent development of themselves first, then the individual employee, the team, and the tribes within the organization. It is about leadership effectiveness, implementing small changes over time. It's about empowering your employees and maintaining a culture of integrity. It is not a task, or a project, or a product - it is a lifestyle. I would venture to say that the addition of the Kaizen philosophy, whether you call it Kaizen, personal development, leadership development, or anything else, is semantics at best. It's not about what you call it; it's about what you do. It's the commitment to improve continuously, one small step at a time. One slight breeze of the butterfly can have profound effects.

I like the definition, "change for the good." As a leader, every day you wake up, every move you make, every breath you take should be a change for the better.

Are you leading yourself and your healthcare team with the philosophy of continuous and ongoing change for the better?

Are you motioning for and with your employees to make some small incremental steps towards improvement?

Do you have a plan? A start of a plan? Thought of a plan?

Thought about thinking about a plan?

Most of you reading this book may have answered 'yes' to the last question.

When you implement small improvements daily, in a small way, it challenges the status quo, causes you to create new habits, and your team to expect more. When you fine-tune the way you live personally and do business professionally, as time moves on, you will see that you will be fine-tuning regularly.

Let's think about this; everything ever created by man started with a thought in someone's mind. The idea then leads to a concept, design, and creation of the 'thing' that was first thought. Your own Kaizen philosophy and attitude must start with an idea in your mind. Make the determination where one small aspect of your life can change today. Instill habits that will focus on your development and effectiveness on others, and your desire and passion for changing. Starting with one small, easy aspect to implement change in your life and your team. Over time, you will see that you created positive results for yourself and your relationships when you look back.

As a manager or director in a memory care organization, think about several ways, concepts, or ideas that you can implement to change the way you serve the patient. Write it down, and let it grow. Visit the vision every day, even for a moment. Plant the seed, water it, and make sure it gets plenty of sunlight.

Book Recommendation

Power of Habits

Learn how to customize your life and your habits. Change the way you operate and start your day. This book changed the way I woke up every day. I began by customizing my mornings to develop this book with just 15 minutes. A 15 minute, or 10 minute or 5 minute change is easy to implement in your lifestyle. I strongly recommend the book P.O.H. - it could change your life.

Kaizen is about small changes involving everyone on your team. It requires persistence and tenacity. The leader needs to be stronger for others who may find themselves pulled into the downward spiral of healthcare compliance, legalities, and insurance fire-fighting. They are walking-the-talk of the vision. They are not walking a trail of outside influences. Their walk will mold the mission and not overcome the vision's adversities or the leader's effectiveness.

Your personal and professional development as a leader is crucial to your team's personal and professional development and its individuals.

Small change point: Often, leaders get caught up pushing important projects aside when the 'seemingly' more critical concept of fire-fighting a compliance or legal issue rears its head. They are then knee-deep in ashes and cinders before realizing that the fire was not the priority they thought it was. The 'fire-fighting' could have been handled by someone else. And now, in choosing to fight that fire themselves, once that fire is extinguished, they have another fire. Choose your fires carefully.

When you become aware of your thoughts and following actions in the advent of an oncoming compliance hurricane, you can stop the automatic urge to run into the fire as leadership personalities tend to do, and be prepared to delegate and move on.

Leader beware of the firefighter in you! He contemplates his next target, his heart racing, sweat at his brow, and shakes in anticipation. Grimacing in amusement as he prepares to wield his water cannon towards the next blaze of potential risk, the spark of possible loss, or the flare of proposed sanctions.

Qualities of a Kaizen Leader:

Effective - The Kaizen leader is an effective leader who does not like waste. They maximize their efforts by focusing on areas of high importance.

In the '*4 Disciplines of Execution*', the authors use the term 'whirlwind' as the large amount of energy you and your team (or organization) use to maintain its current level. The 'whirlwind' makes it hard to execute those things that are of higher importance. The 'whirlwind' is a thieve taking time and energy away from those things that will propel you and your team forward in the care of your patients and families.

Importance is a Priority: They want to choose importance in a way that will lead both their life and their team.

Maximizers: Kaizen leaders are efficient, strategic and maximize their value for the organization and its people.

Collaboration: Kaizen leaders enjoy collaboration to create efficiency, reduce waste, improve learning, and develop powerful teams. They enjoy brainstorming with their team, organizing, ordering priorities, and implementing ideas with their team.

Small Steps: Kaizen leaders prefer small improvements over big jumps in processes and individual and team development.

Training and Education: Kaizen leaders realize that front-line employees should learn practical problem-solving skills through training, education, and learning.

Empowering: Kaizen leaders enjoy empowering individual and team leadership opportunities.

Crystal: Kaizen leaders are clear and concise in their communication. They make sure they understand the team, and each player seeks to be sure that the overall vision and message is crystal clear to everyone.

Elephants are a Staple: As I tell my children, Kaizen leaders enjoy the daily supplementation of elephants' tidbits as part of their daily routine.

Effective – The Fifth Strategy

> *"Leadership is doing the right things, and Management is doing things right."*
> *- Peter Drucker.*

When I was in the systems consulting business and then the fitness business, I was always trying to do more with less. I tried to cram in as many things as possible in my morning routines in a few hours. I loved saying, "I do more before 9 am than most people do the whole week". I think that came from an Army slogan. Well, I used to brag about that for years. In hindsight, I was trying to go as fast as I could in one direction. In my maturity, I realized that life does not travel in a straight line. A single simple day does not travel in a straight line.

I thought that the best way to 6 was 1+2+3. Archimedes was my hero because I saw life as a straight and simple equation. Archimedes is the one who stated that the shortest distance between two points is a straight line. He talked about math and geometry, and I am sure a few other things past my comprehension. But that rule does not apply in life.

It wasn't until many years later that I understood the power of effectiveness. Less is more, doing what's right and good is more important, and quality is better than quantity. Significantly, and most importantly, in relationships.

Putting effectiveness first is crucial to the power and passion in your relationships. Employees will find the source of their motivation in the quality of the communication and the leader's heart - in you.

Attention managers, directors, case managers, and supervisors (and C-level suite); if you are micro-managing your staff, you focus on quantity - not quality.

Stop, it hurts. It's painful and not productive. It does not focus on the relationship but the work. You can concentrate on the work and the quality of the connection simultaneously if you put the relationship first. Focus on every single relationship, every single communication, in your employees, and not the checklist.

As a senior care administrator at any level, learning to be an effective leader is one of the best ways to create a positive, flourishing culture with those you serve.

Let's first define effectiveness.

The primary focus of effectiveness is on the results. It is aligned with leadership. It looks at the process and results from a 30,000-foot view and is more relationship-focused, centered on how people function together. Effective leaders are concerned with the individual's motivation, the communication within teams, and each project's mission. Coloring outside the lines is encouraged. Timelines are not as important as looking at the result - the vision. Managers, directors, team leaders, and case managers can all be effective leaders. Remember, the manager is a title - being a leader is a function of who you are in your management role.

Let's look at efficiency. Efficiency is about performance and can be noted as a management function. Its daily productivity is task-focused, breaking projects down to their minute detail. Its focus is on the reduction of waste, whether it be time, productivity, or resources. Efficient management is focused on fast and immediate results with shorter timelines. Coloring outside the lines is not encouraged - it's considered a waste of time and resources.

Efficiency is similar to looking at the miles per gallon as the primary focus of traveling from one place to another, while leadership may focus on the journey. Efficiency is trying to fit as many clowns as possible into a Volkswagen bug with little concern about breathing space. Leaders may want to make sure that the clowns arrive alive and cheerful.

Dementia care management is centered on the efficiency of resources. Compliance, insurance, and regulations are all balanced on the formulas of efficiency. Dementia care leaders should be focused on delivering the vision and the journey with the employees. Together, leadership and management should be concerned with 'doing the right things, right.'

Efficiency and effectiveness are both important and required for a high quality, high-performance healthcare organization. Those companies that lack effective leadership have high turnover, poor communication, lack of team cohesiveness, focusing on priorities, and not what's important.

It's the difference between being employee-centered or compliance-focused. It's about living the vision or the 'this is how the company does it' mentality by being effective and focusing on quality or being efficient and focusing on quantity. As I stated earlier, you need both.

That does not mean that the numbers, compliance, and the rules and regulations do not count. They do matter and are essential. They are not the most important, and very seldom do they prioritize the customer and the employee.

It's easier in the compliance centered, fire-fighting industry to be focused on efficiency, even at the leadership level. When the leadership is focused on management functions such as efficiency, they sacrifice quality and growth, the individual, the teams, and the final product.

The leader knows how and when to use effectiveness and efficiency, in the right way, at the right time, with the right people - the right way.

Effective leaders:

Are Challenged: Effective leaders see the daily challenges answered with a focus on the vision.

Hire Smart: Effective leaders hire those that are smarter and better than they are in specific areas. They seek out those they can trust. They do not hire a warm body to fill an empty seat based on a resume alone.

Have a High Emotional I.Q.: According to the Harvard Business Review, emotional intelligence is a skill necessary for a leader to be effective. If they don't have the skills, they work on them every day.

Are Empathetic: Effective leaders master the management of their relationships in a positive and nurturing way.

Have a High Standard of Excellence: Effective leaders intentionally set examples, allow themselves to be vulnerable, take appropriate risks, and empower their teams.

Motivate and Inspire: Effective leaders are challenged and determined to see the value in others.

Do What is Good and Right: Effective leaders believe in what is good and what is right and that these qualities can be found in others.

Have a Clear Vision: Points the team and its' members in the same direction, working towards the same goal providing a clear vision for the team, department, or project.

Empowering – The Sixth Strategy

> *"Do not follow where the path may lead.*
> *Go instead, where there is no path and leave a trail."*
> *Muriel Strode*

I had visited a family home the day before the patient moved into an assisted living facility. Joe was an 85-year-old man with dementia. He was in his later stages and had just been admitted to hospice care. Joe's children promised him that they would keep him home no matter what, "they would find a way" was what Jennie, the youngest daughter, cried. Yet, little did they realize how difficult it would be to care for their father, maintain their own families, live out of state, and keep their jobs. It was a challenge that was facing families daily.

I visited Joe a week after the move. It was clear that Joe was anxious. He was confused and didn't know why. Joe thought he was at work and was waiting for the closing bell so he could go home. He couldn't sleep at night because he could not find his bed and had been missing his wife. He told me there was 'no cuddling'. During the day Joe was walking around asking for the bus stop.

Maria was an aide at the facility who quickly fell in love with Joe. As soon as she came to work, Joe was the first person she visited. She told me that she somehow felt his frustration. Maria was a good aide - she was given a schedule and did what she was told. However, she felt as if the management was not listening to her advice on some of the patients' care.

But when it came to Joe, she felt something different. She saw him differently and was filled with emotion and compassion when it came to his care. "I can't sit and let him be anxious the way he is. I must do something." She had two ideas that would help Joe, but both were against policy. First, she thought that Joe should have his own bed - yet the facility's policies did not allow for outside beds because they had a major bed bug infestation several years ago.

The second recommendation was that Joe could use a body pillow to hug and hold. She knew this was against the rules, so she did not recommend it for fear of being reprimanded. Maria called me aside. Together we decided that we should talk at length after work. We met at a

Starbucks to talk. I offered Maria some suggestions to re-think her priorities. Encouraging and enforcing the notion that doing what is right and good will always benefit the people involved - especially the patient. It was clear that Maria had suppressed her priorities for the rules and regulations of the facility. She felt that no one was listening, and as a result, after many years, she exclaimed, 'kept quiet and did what was told'.

I left Maria, hoping that she was going to do the right thing. A week later, I visited the facility where I bumped into Maria's manager - Angelica. She stated, "Chris, I understand you had a private conversation with Maria. Can we talk in my office?". "Of course," I said, "Can you give me ten minutes?". I checked in with one of my team members and met Angelica in her office. I was waiting for some kind of complaint and finger-pointing. Instead, Angelica stated she was 'ecstatic' at what has transpired in the past week.

Angelica explained that she had been in the position for just over a year, and before that, over the past three years, the facility could not keep a manager for more than six months. "It was an uphill battle, but it's getting better," she added. She further explained some of the communication issues and challenges in getting the front-line staff to open up and talk. "After speaking with Maria, I realized that they (*the staff*) did not feel heard and empowered."

She explained that Maria asked for a meeting to discuss the facility's rules and how she wanted permission to change the rules to accommodate the patients' needs. Angelica stated, "She was so nervous and so gentle about the request that I could barely hear her speak. But after she explained in detail her desires to serve Joe, I said, yes - do it. I told her this is now her project to own it and get it done."

Angelica stated that Maria's tone, body posture, and facial expression completely transformed before her eyes. You could see the joy coming out of her when she received the permission needed to do what was required to care for the patients - especially Joe.

As a result of Maria's courage, the rules of the patient's furniture have been reversed, and many rules and regulations restricting the effectiveness of the front-line staff were reversed. Angelica stated she is getting the front-line staff involved in the process; she is listening and taking their advice seriously. As a result, Maria was asked to take on as a being the liaison between the front-line staff and management.

Maria now walks with her head high and a spring in her step, knowing that taking action and doing what was important for the patient does offer many people benefits. She has more confidence in her employer and management.

Maria took charge of coordinating with Joe's family to move his bed from their home to the facility. Maria asked the family for permission to purchase a body pillow for Joe. She later returned to the facility that evening on her own time to tuck Joe in and give him the gift of the body pillow. For the first time in weeks, Joe slept all night in his bed - 'cuddling' his new pillow.

Empowering is giving power to the employees, especially the front-line staff. Empowering is assigning them the rights to make the decisions and perform the tasks necessary that need to be made when they need to be made for the sole benefit of the patient and family.

On the other hand, delegation is the manager making the decisions on the tasks that need to be done and assigning those tasks to individuals. It's a to-do list of items with employees' names next to each item. You hand out the list, the employee looks for their name, and completes the task. This process is not empowering, yet it does have its place.

When it comes to empowering, the leader seeks to convey what needs to be accomplished. In a shared tone, an agreement is made on how the project's goals should be achieved. Delegation is more a manager or supervisor function, whereas empowering is a leadership and vision function.

Empowering is a big deal, a considerable aspect of corporate leadership. One of those aspects of an organization that is part of the walk-the-talk, action-oriented, watch how I do leadership. When it's done well, it weaves itself in and out of the organization's culture and sub-cultures. It weaves a tapestry that ties together a sense of belonging and purpose within the employee base. It makes for a strong foundation. But there is something inherent in empowering leaders that is more than the concept of sharing, more than getting the employees involved. It's the heart.

This whole book is about the heart of the leader. It's about those thoughts that are in the deepest parts of the leaders' psyche. It's their emotional and spiritual connection. It's the compassion and empathy that brings passion and fire. That's what comes first - an empowering leadership attitude. It comes before any pen touches paper, any word meets an ear, and before any concept becomes a reality. The heart of the leader comes first and foremost.

From the heart of empowerment is a servant leader's heart. It desires to put others first, share ideas and concepts, give power away, and allow decisions to be made by caring for the patients and families. The words empower, servant, and share are always used in concert when discussing leadership.

Empowering leaders consistently grow and develop themselves and others - never stagnating or staying the same. They engage and support vertical and horizontal thinking and learning. They are always looking for suggestions, meeting problems as challenges, and seeking to solve them with a win-win attitude.

Empowering leaders love a big box of crayons. Crayons are colorful and bold. The bigger the box, the more variety - yet leaders can also work with a small box of crayons just as well. Since leaders are out of the box thinkers, they look for people who can also 'color outside the lines'. In the healthcare world, many lines are drawn. From compliance, insurance, and government regulations, employees are challenged to always stay within the lines.

However, many decisions can be made when we go outside the lines. I don't mean to break the rules intentionally - rules are essential and needed to run and operate an organization correctly. And most of those rules are at a minimum, minimum required standards that need to be practiced. However, thinking or coloring outside the lines allows employees to discover new and better ways of caring and loving their patients and families.

There is a word you do not see in compliance, insurance, or government rulebooks. That word is love. Love has no boundaries - so how can we be expected to serve with love and compassion within a compliance centered world. We can't. Your employees must be given the authority to color outside the lines. They must be allowed to love and care for those they are commissioned to serve. They should be allowed to express the joy and happiness of sharing the love as an integral part of their empowerment.

Empowering leaders share power and responsibility first. They must then reciprocate and get feedback on new ideas and concepts and the joy and happiness it takes from caring for others. This one factor is the most critical in empowering others - listening to joy. When someone shares the joy in the love they have given, they get to relive that joy again and again. It begins to grow and develop not only in those that share but with those that are listening. Vicarious communication is a communicable aspect of empowering that allows it to seed in the hearts of others. When you walk-the-talk, you spread the sunshine and water the seed - and watch it grow.

Let me make one mention here - empowering leaders do not micro-manage. Micro-managing is anti-empowering. It is a control and insecurity issue by poor management. An ineffective management style that crushes employees. It makes them stifle and stop, forcing them to perform at their minimum.

Sidebar:
Remember, in the chapter on passion, I suggested changing the word 'problem' to 'challenge'? Well, here's another word to change.
Ever notice how people will say they are nervous when they do public speaking or enter an event or contest, even though they are passionate about a task?
Simon Sinek suggests changing the word 'nervous' to 'excited.' You will notice that the word 'excited' redefines and carries a whole new meaning and perception in how you feel about what is happening within you.

A compliance-driven individual is not a leader but a manager. Compliance, insurance, and regulation-based healthcare organizations do the following, in most part, unintentionally:

1. Restrict empowerment
2. Restrict the creativity of employees
3. Restrict opportunities for growth
4. Enforce coloring inside the lines as the only acceptable behavior
5. Usually, gives only one color to crayon work with - black.
6. React to problems instead of being proactive to challenges
7. Lacks a trusting atmosphere

8. Promotes teams working in silos and encourages lone wolf mentality (see Strategy 7 - Tribe)

Empowering leaders:

Mentor: Empowering leaders create and maintain a mentoring program that includes all members of the organization.

Promote Growth: Empowering leaders promote growth and productivity in their teams and the individual.

Challenge: Empowering leaders place individuals in positions where they are challenged and supported. They seek out opportunities to serve and support.

Offer a Winning Atmosphere: Empowering leaders support small incremental wins and support failures as part of growth and development.

'Stay the Sword': Empowering leaders withhold judgment, supporting self-evaluation and self-confidence. They don't shoot first and ask questions later.

Encouraging: Empowering leaders encourage ideas and communication, enlisting proactive listening in teams and individuals.

Tribe, Teams, and Wolves – The Seventh Strategy

> *"I invite everyone to choose forgiveness rather than division, teamwork over personal ambition." - Jean-Francois Cope.*

A fighter pilot named Charles Plumb was shot down by a missile on his 75th mission while flying over Vietnam. He ejected from his plane, captured by the Vietnamese, and held captive for six years. One day after his release, a man came up to him and said, "You are Charles Plumb, aren't you?" Charles looked at him in shock and replied, "How did you know that?" The man said, "I packed your parachute." Plumb was surprised and, in gratitude, said, "I guess it worked?" Plumb couldn't stop thinking about the man that packed his parachute. Charles thought of the countless hours that man had packed each parachute, knowing he had someone's life in his hands.

Each of you who are managers, directors, or leaders in the home care, hospice, or assisted living depends on others to do your job well. In this respect, there are two types of people, those who realize their interdependence on others and those who don't - those who don't are the 'lone wolves' bred by the compliance and regulatory-centered organizations.

As a hospice chaplain, I depended on communication with the nurses, aides, social workers, and volunteers to help me get a full picture of how to serve the patient and families best. In most cases, the turnover rate was so high, and the focus on compliance was so intense on appropriate documentation and timeliness that contact was few and far between. There was not an intended plan of communication within the team. It was only with individuals, talking with one another. Not together as a team.

My mode of communication is always proactive, communicating with those I work with before any need arises. I usually place in the subject of an email with an "F.Y.I.," just if they need information regarding a patient. On several occasions, I have been met with hostility from my teammates as the intended recipient did not understand the purpose of the 'heads up.' I was once told by a manager, "since there was no fire, there was no need to have a bucket of water at their side." I was told to "just do spiritual things and let everyone else do their jobs."

Of course, I did what was right, and on more than many occasions, the information proved fruitful albeit unrecognized - but hey, just as long as the patient benefited - right? I don't think so. You see, in weaving a tapestry of teamwork, we must first be aware that there are many threads interwoven for a specific purpose. Without appropriate team support, which brings many colors of life, compassion, relationships, and, dare I say, love, we weave a dark piece of cloth that keeps the patient warm but not well served.

We can weave our tapestry and do a good job, or we can do a great job well. The quality of our relationships will dictate the quality of service received by our patients. Since this chapter is focused on teamwork, let's first start by clearly defining a few things related to serving together for the benefit of the patients and families.

Tribes - Are a group of multiple teams working for the same or similar area, department, project, or a specific group of patients and families. Think region or for small companies that focus on one area, it could be the whole company.

Teams - Are a part of a tribe. They are a small group of people tasked with caring for patients and families in a healthcare environment. The team can be classified according to a project, or maybe a disease or condition. Teams most likely have between eight and twelve employees as members.

Silos - groups of individuals within the organization, tribe, or team that feel they do not need to share information. They work as independent units appearing detached from the vision. Silos are a product of the senior care sector and how it works, and this is based on a lot of my own experience. Compliance driven organizations produce silos.

Lone Wolves - These individuals appear to be 'good' team members and are good at deception. They thrive in units that do not naturally collaborate, such as interdisciplinary teams. Lone wolves thrive in groups functioning well on the surface where their influence is horizontal, not vertical, and deep. Lone wolves only share information if it's necessary and required. They don't freely offer support unless it's 'part of the job'. Lone wolves say things like, "Let me do my job," or "that's your job responsibility, not mine." They may get involved in fellow team members' responsibilities to increase their stature or obtain recognition.

In the healthcare field, by design, we work in teams. Sometimes those teams or their members do not comprehend how they relate to other teams within the organization. As the only team member with a specialty, individuals are naturally singled out as the 'best' or 'most qualified' to belong on the team, adding to the silo or lone wolf concept. The review process is focused on how you did, against yourself, not necessarily how well you collaborated and shared with your fellow team members.

For lone wolves in silos, synergy and collaboration are not words in their vocabulary. Their natural tendency is apathetic and passive. Their future is seen as how quickly and efficiently they can advance the corporate ladder, grow in their careers, or it can be as simple as self-recognition.

It takes pro-active leadership with a passion for serving others to create and maintain a high-performance team. The leader has to overcome the natural tendency for team members to act as a lone wolf mentality within the silo. It's the manager, director, or individual on the front lines with the right attitude towards success in relationships who cultivates the gift of a leader's heart.

As a leader, to have a vision, you need a team of individuals who collaborate with a common goal. Knowing your team, and even more importantly, knowing where you are within the structure of the tribe, is just as important as conveying the vision to your team. Whether you are a manager, director, or team lead, you have the responsibility to create and maintain a sharing, collaborative mentality with the members. Dissuading the silo and lone wolf mentality is needed to take on a clear vision for the organization and the team. It's important to recognize the teams' individuals in their participation and collaborative efforts by including a ceremony and celebration of the team.

The title of this book is the 'real' question each team member must be able to answer:
Who am I? And What am I doing here?
Can your team members answer those two questions?
Do they know the team vision and mission, the values and goals?
Are they recognized for who they are within the team?
Additionally, are they recognized for how they collaborate with the other team members?
Do they know their individual as well as team goals and action items?
And

Do they understand how each team member is aligned with the others?
Is their caring as well as sharing?
Is their compassion within the team?
Compassion is one of those values that, when shared, expands exponentially. And when that happens, there is more for families and patients.

Qualities of a Team-Centered Leader:

Walk the talk: Team centered leaders reflect their team's image as that team reflects their leadership. This reflection goes hand in hand with walking the talk. Be the person and the leader you want to be in the future and begin practicing those behaviors now. Your team will reflect your leadership.

Color Outside the Lines: Team centered leaders give their team a big box of crayons and color outside the lines. Team centered leaders watch where the team creates that image of the collaboration of a high-performance team.

Compassion: Team centered leaders create an environment of compassion and empathy in a person-centered team. Team leaders care about their people and put the individuals and the team first.

Perseverance: Team-centered leaders know that with perseverance and determinism, the team's colors will change and they may need a new box of crayons. In time, they will become more patient-centered, caring, and respectful - first to each other and, as a result, better serve the patients and families.

Appendix

Recommended Leadership Books

"Not all readers are leaders, but all leaders are readers." - Harry Truman.

Below are just a few books that I have read and studied over the years - most of them two and three times. Leadership is a daily practice; reading is step one... the rest includes implementation and inspiration.

Suggestion:

- Take one book - master it, don't just read it.
- Move on.
- Start a book club with other leaders, or start a book club with some of your managers and aspiring leaders.
- One hour a week, one chapter a week, and share - do it over breakfast. I promise you won't regret it.

Good to Great, Why Some Companies Make the Leap, and Others Don't - **Jim Collins**

I list this one first because I think it could significantly impact how you do leadership. I read this book at least five times over the past ten years, and I think I will 'listen' to it again. Buy the book and the audio.

The book took five years of research and writing to put together. Jim Collins looked at eleven companies that were poor to average and then had what appears to have been a sudden success.

They learned that there was no sudden success and that it took simple vision and goals over time that lead to sustainable success.

Strong servant leadership does not happen overnight. It takes a proactive approach to the service of others. It's intentional leadership that sustains long-term success.

Leading at a Higher Level **- Ken Blanchard**

Ken Blanchard is my all-time favorite author and inspiration. I enjoyed every one of his books that I read, but I think this is probably my best.

It's about world-class leadership. It's about vision, goals, who you are, where you (and your organization) are going, and making sure everyone knows. It encompasses the teachings of Situational Leadership in leading yourself, individuals, teams, and the organization.

Its concepts can be applied to all areas of your life, personal and professional.

A must-read...

Thinking for a Change, 11 Ways Highly Successful People Approach Work **- John Maxwell**

A simple and easy read will teach you how to think in ways that will keep you ahead and make a difference in your life and others' lives.

Take each chapter as a lesson, read it, reread it, then apply the principles in your life. Master them, then go to the next chapter.

Resonant Leadership - **Richard Boyatzis and Annie McKee**

These two authors wrote Primal Leadership, a good book as well. Although not on my list, it belongs on your bookshelf (after you read it, of course).

This book is about the heart of leadership, with wisdom and practical applications. It's about empathy, hope, and compassion in the business world.

Shout out to Richard Boyatzis, who endorsed this book! Thanks Richard!

The Heart of a Leader, Insights on the Art of Influence - **Ken Blanchard**

The is a great little book that you can keep on your desk. Open it up once in a while to get tidbits of powerful information, most of which you can implement immediately.

Find tips like the one on page 20, 'When you stop growing, you stop learning,' or how about this one, which directly corresponds to growing and developing your people, it's on page 84; "People without information cannot act responsibly. People with information are compelled to act responsibly."

The Leadership Challenge - **Kouzes and Posner**

This is a book to study and not over the weekend. It's a big book of over 400 pages, and if you feel inclined, there is an accompanying workbook. I always wanted to make this book a workshop, maybe a 'book club' item.

Kouzes and Posner analyze and break down what the most inspiring leaders do so that you can do the same and achieve the same results. They have developed a leadership model that consists of what they call the Five Practices of Exemplary Leadership®.

The 5 Languages of Appreciation in the Workplace, Empowering Organizations by Encouraging People **- Gary Chapman and Paul White**

You will see this again in my world, especially if I can bring this powerful book to your workplace.

It's about influences through appreciation and valuing others - your employees. It takes a proactive, conscious effort, but it pays off big time. This book equips you with the tools you need to create an atmosphere of appreciation.

Easy to read, easy to implement, and easy to share. The corresponding website offers online workshops.

www.appreciationatwork.com

Leading Change **- John P. Kotter**

I studied this book and the '*Leadership Challenge*' when I started my Masters in Strategic Communication and Leadership at Seton Hall University. I never finished my Masters; however, I did learn a huge amount from this book. It's about culture and how to change the culture. Like everything else I read about leadership, change is not overnight - it takes time, persistence, and determination.

The biggest thing I learned is that you cannot get past the point that a leader's most important task is to have a vision and help others "buy into" that vision. Operative words are 'buy into.' Without the 'buy-in,' you can't move forward.

21 Laws of Leadership, Follow Them and People Will Follow You - **John Maxwell**

Simple, easy to read, easy to understand.

Take a law, read it, implement it. Once you master it, read the next law. It takes time, so make it a challenge. One week, master one law.

Let me know how you do.

Those were a few of the top books that I refer to over the years.

Here are a few more:

- *Servant Leadership: A Journey into the Nature of Legitimate Power and Greatness* – 25th Anniversary Edition by Robert Greenleaf

- *Leaders Eat Last: Why Some Teams Pull Together, and Others Don't* – by Simon Sinek.

- *The Servant Leader: How to Build a Creative Team, Develop Great Morale, and Improve Bottom-Line Performance* – by James A. Autry

- *Leadership Is an Art* – by Max De Pree

- *The World's Most Powerful Leadership Principle: How to Become a Servant Leader* – by James Hunter

- *Multipliers* – by Liz Wiseman

- *The Secret* – by Ken Blanchard and Mark Miller

As I mentioned earlier, all of the leadership books I read all take time. They take an intentional, proactive approach to implementing change in your life and the lives of others. And since we are in the dementia care service field, we have an internal compass that points us to serve others. Together, we have a passion and desire to share and serve.

Leadership starts with you first, and it starts with sharing your growth and development with others. Learning to be a passionate servant leader is a lifelong process. Even if you stop intentionally teaching yourself, you will always be learning.

Don't Forget the Elephant.

We have all heard the sayings, 'patience is a virtue.' And that is true, but patience does not lead to success in any area. You must be proactive in your journey to serve.

I have mentioned this quote before, but I use it so much that I wanted to share it again.

I am reminded of a quip that I share with my children and has become a personal mantra. When I want to remind myself, my children, or some people in my business world, I say, "don't forget the elephant' and they know what I mean.

So here it is:

How do you eat an elephant? It can become a daunting task, and if you think about it, it could make one very anxious and overwhelmed.

Well, I say, one bite at a time.

So, I say to you in your quest to becoming a better, smarter, and compassionate leader,

'don't forget the elephant.'

Are you a leader?

> *"If your actions inspire others to dream more, learn more, do more, and become more, you are a leader."* - John Quincy Adams.

The following are a few questions that can help you define who you are and help you put together a list of skills to become a better leader.

Are you someone who enjoys creating something new from nothing?

Do you see problems as challenges and opportunities?

Are you proactive, or do you wait for something to happen even if you see it coming?

Do you want to make a change for the better of others?

Do you think of your team and the members of your team first?

Do you have skills and qualities such as patience, active listening, empathy, positivity, reliability, and team building? If not, are you working on them?

How do you manage conflict in the workplace, and can you negotiate without creating anxiety?

Do you look at vision and goals as a priority or your 'to-do' list?

Do you have a strategic plan for your team or department?

Here are two more questions that will lead you to two assessments that I believe are helpful if you work on them daily.

Do you know your emotional I.Q.?

Search for the 'E.Q. Test' by Daniel Goleman, author of the bestselling book in 1995: Emotional Intelligence.

Do you see yourself in a vocation or a job?

Certain gifts and strengths will lend themselves to an individual who has a natural tendency to enjoy this as a vocation instead of a job. It's what is in the character and personality of the individual. It's not like a skill that can be learned and practiced.

First, what's the difference between job and vocation. Well, **this is my definition:**

- Vocation is a passion - A job is indifference or detachment.
- Vocation is living a dream - A job is dreaming of the end of the day.
- Vocation is what you believe is your calling - A job is just a 'thing you do.'

In a vocation, you desire to learn more, understand more, gain more knowledge, and forge relationships.

A vocation is where you have more than others, and you have a burning desire to share it for the benefit of others.

Gifts

As I just stated, vocation is a calling. With a calling, there is the assumption that you have a gift or gifts to assist you in that calling. Many gifts in many combinations can support your calling as an expert in dementia care operations:

- **Administration** - the captain who steers the ship
- **Encouragement** - to lift others, encourage, and strengthen
- **Giving** - this is self-explanatory - it is the gift to provide without expectations or pretense
- **Leadership** - caring for others, to lead, assist and protect
- **Mercy** - to be patient and compassionate towards others
- **Shepherd** - servants to their people, relationships, in this case - patients and families
- **Service** - care for others that will benefit others without recognition
- **Teaching** - teach, instruct, explain, and expound

It is a combination, usually of two or more gifts that will allow you to use those gifts to serve others. This is not a comprehensive list of gifts. These are gifts that I see in myself and others I have worked with in a similar capacity.

Strengths

There are the gifts, which might be likened to a role or title - but not really - let me explain. Let's look at it this way. Your official title would be, for example, Director of Operations of Dementia Care. Your role is to create and manage the process of bringing dementia care training to the employees and understanding of dementia to the community, patients, and families (that's it in a nutshell, of course, there is much more.)

My leadership, administration, shepherding, and teaching gifts help me take responsibility and tap into internal resources to be that leader, director (or manager).

Your strengths are the toolbox. They are the hammer and chisel, the scalpel and forceps, or the podium and script.

Clifton Strengths Finder is a powerful and useful assessment tool to help you understand your strengths. I have seen this in myself and others. When you discover your strengths (and gifts), you begin to notice why you did what you did in the past and how you can use those strengths with confidence in your future. When you become aware of your strengths, you naturally become passionate about your new knowledge and confidence.

My strategic, connectedness, arranger, and maximizer strengths allow me to quickly and easily see how complex plans come together. With a natural 30,000-foot view, I can innately see the connection between people, relationships, places, and things. With that view, I can arrange for an effective outcome for the organization, the process, and most importantly, the people I serve.

To see the bigger picture, using myself as an example, my gifts of leadership, administration, shepherding, and teaching with my toolbox of strengths of strategic, connectedness, arranger and maximizer come together to serve best the needs of the organization and the needs of the patient and families (as well as community). When I am mindful of the gifts and strengths in action, there is a passion that drives me towards a win-win-win situation for all my relationships.

Do you know your strengths?

www.Gallup.com/cliftonstrengths

Strategic Planning

Search the internet for strategic plans. With some creativity and determination, a simple vision, mission, and strategic planning session can begin the process of tying the team together. You will find that the session will be informative and enjoyable for everyone.

The WAG - Woodbridge Advisory Group

Mastermind Roundtable and Peer-to-Peer Advisory Groups
A Monthly Roundtable For Senior Care Administrators, Directors and Managers

Whether you are operating an Assisted Living Facility, Memory Care Unit, Hospice, Home Care, or Adult Day Care, being successful doesn't require you to be stressed and overwhelmed.

Turn your hard work into a rewarding experience. Join other dementia care managers and directors like you who have taken the right actions to grow themselves, their teams, and the organization by engaging in the powerful mastermind group principle of peer-driven success.

This senior healthcare community provides collaborative, practical, solution-oriented discussions to addresses the most challenging problems we all face.

Ensure your organization's predictable growth and success. Woodbridge Advisory Group's, Mastermind Peer-Advisory groups provide a systematic way to inject new ideas, viewpoints, and perspectives. It operates as an informal board of directors, coach, and peer advisory group – with much less demand on your time and financial resources.

Visit the WAG at:
www.WAG.TheWellspringSenior.com

Dementia Leadership Certifications,

Dementia Friendly Facilities™

And Live Certification™

Coming 2021

- Live Certification™

- Dementia Appreciation Support Certification Workshop

- Dementia Care Leader Certification

- Senior Care Leader Certification

- Board Certified Dementia Care Leader

Visit:

www.TheWellspringSenior.com

Some of the Stories Behind the Story

"It always seems impossible until it's done." - Nelson Mandela.

All my life, I have been interested in leadership development. Since the mid-nineties', that's 1990's, I have absorbed dozens of books, attended seminars, workshops, and classes wherever and whenever I could. I became certified as a leadership consultant, created and facilitated retreats, consulted, and coached.

The more I learned, the more I realized that I became more passionate in two areas of leadership development. The first is called servant leadership - it differs from other leadership, especially that of change leadership, which I believe may be focused at a much higher organizational hierarchy level.

For me, servant leadership is more about caring for and serving the people. It's about being close to the people, both the employees and the clients - in our case, the patients and the families. As you will see, the best way to get to the patient, to offer patient-centered care is through the employees.

Love your patients by first loving your employees - I think that should be my philosophy. What do you think?

The second area of focus is on the personal development of the leader. Some call it personal leadership development. This was a challenging area for me because when I started resurrecting this focus for business leaders, I was shunned by my church. They believed that to focus on self was a sin of pride. Save that journey for some other tale. I no longer belong to that church.

My belief is, and I find others believe this as well, is to become an effective leader, servant, change, transformational, or any other type, one must know about ourselves first. This lifelong journey must start with a commitment to excel in self to serve others. Not to serve oneself - herein lies the sin.

As I progressed in my career journey, I moved into the healthcare field as a hospice chaplain. I immediately knew I was different from the comments made during the interviews. Two directors from two hospice organizations, five years apart, both said, "You're different than any other chaplain - you have a unique set of skills." That's how I knew I was different.

I was and still am focused on how people serve, on the effectiveness and quality of the care. I was always asking, "Can they (those that are serving at all levels) do a better job at that moment, and can we learn from each other?" Over time, I became keenly interested in the dementia field. Those 'friends' with dementia in assisted living facilities and home care were not yet at the hospice level.

In almost every facility I visited, which was dozens of facilities over the years, I noticed that dementia care was poor for most facilities. This is my rating, and the care was not inadequate - just poor based on my standards. Additionally, I noticed that the only organizations offering higher quality care were charging 200 -300% more than the national average. This, to me, was an atrocity.

Yet, increasing the organization's learning does not cost that much, and, over time, training becomes a valued investment. Ah! Hence my vision, or at least the start of it. Years of watching, observing, learning, assessing, and getting trained and certified, I realized the following:

1. We (the healthcare field) are not ready for the ongoing wave of our ' friends' with dementia. That wave is preceded by the 'Silver Tsunami" of the Baby Boomers.

2. We do not have the leadership, the servant leadership, to implement a strategy of ongoing, regular, and consistent development for those individuals at the front and on the supportive lines.

3. It's not that hard. It's very easy.

Hence, this book started as a mind dump. Part one was written in a weekend and modified throughout a couple of months, adding part two.

With the research I was doing, I realized that something had to be done. I created the Dementia Friendly Facility™ certification as an easily accessible and highly affordable 'live' dementia care certification process. My goal was to make it affordable for the individual employee as well as the organization. Why? In my view, the cost of education and training should not be a hindrance to quality service to the individual patient and family.

Over time, I believe assisted living facilities, home care, and hospice organizations can be fully trained to understand, appreciate, and care for our 'friends' with dementia in a compassionate and supportive manner.

About the Main Characters: Maxx, Duke, Maggie, and Ginger

These characters and their personalities were taken from my pets.

Maxx - a Landseer Newfoundland

Duke - a black Labrador Retriever

Maggie - a black and white Great Dane and rescue

Ginger - an orange female Tabby

And the other character is Zeppoles. Yes, Zepploes is a character!

One day I was watching a show that was taking place in Little Italy during the San Gennaro Festival. Since I lived and worked in New York during my younger days, I visited Little Italy and frequently attended the festivals.

Zeppoles was always something that we had to bring home for the rest of the family. If you have never had a Zeppole...well, Zepps is a deep-fried ball of dough with a splash of sugar. It's like a warm cloud of sunshine.

It is said, "Naples invented zeppole, and all Italians licked their fingers."

So there you go, some of the story behind the story... and in writing these last words on this last page, may I add this prayer to you:

May the Lord bless you and keep you and always shine His face upon you...

Now, go get a Zepp...!

Final Thoughts

"Whenever you have taken up work in hand, you must see it to the finish. That is the ultimate secret of success. Never, never, never give up!" - Dada Vaswani.

My final note is directed to you, the managers, team leaders, supervisors, case managers, and those who aspire to influence others in the field of dementia care (and senior care). This book is about you and for you. You have the opportunity, the position, the role, and the power to empower and enrich the lives of others.

My advice is to take one small item that was the most appealing from one chapter and make one small change in your life every day. And add to that change ways where you can help someone else for the better and the good, for their good, for the good of the patient - not for your good - although that will be a reward in the journey.

- Being a leader is a skill, as well as a gift. And like any skill (and gift), it must be maintained, or it will be lost. The adage if you don't use it, you lose it, is true.
- Being a leader is intentional - you must plan to lead and lead the plan.
- Being a leader is not going just to happen.
- Being a leader in dementia care starts with planting the seed of care and compassion.
- It must be created and cultivated - it takes time. It takes people. It takes lives.
- Being a leader in dementia care is not about the patient - well, maybe it is. But it is getting to the patients with your service to the employees. You cannot get to the patient without the employees - first.

If you have read this far, you already know that I place high importance on the employees first. I said it before, and I have no regrets in repeating it, and out loud,

'You Must Love Your Employees'.

I didn't mention this yet, but I will here. I didn't say you have to like your employees, but you must love them and what they do. Each one of them desires to serve others, yet each one conveys that desire in different ways. And even though we may disagree on how they manage their day-to-day, loving them is different. Loving them for who they are, for their passion and desire is what is essential. The liking part is about the skill.

This is how I look at it, and it helps me - 'Love' is about passion, 'like' is about the skill. We can grow to 'like' someone if we have a desire to be compassionate and understanding. Love is the passion that gets us there.

If we realize that the patient is always the priority and the employees are always the most important, we can be a step ahead in serving. Keep in mind; it's more involved than words on a paper. It requires you, the leader, to walk the talk and act as if the camera is always on you. Being a leader is leading, especially when no one is watching. It's not only about being the frontman, but it's about being the fall guy, with grace and humility.

Being a leader and a manager in dementia care is hard - real hard. The rules and regulations are always changing, always correcting, always judging, and I agree - it's a necessary evil. But like traffic lights and crosswalks, there is a time and place for each. Without them, people will get hurt. They will have trouble getting to and from their daily destinations, being unable to accomplish the organization's goals in the proper care of the individual - whether it's the employee or the patient.

Being a leader is about cultivating and learning. I love learning. I enjoy the process so much that I get too involved and get burned out. Yet I still enjoy it, and I enjoy spreading that learning with others whenever I can. I think the one thing I enjoy more than learning is watching the light bulbs come on when people learn something new and understand how they can apply that learning in their lives - especially with their team or patients.

I love the learning so much that I am creating a certification and training program for those frontline staff who desire to be leaders caring for people with dementia at the same time of publication as the publications of this book. I intend to make it easy to access, easy to acquire, and easy to maintain

Most importantly, let me finish by saying always strive to be your best by doing your best and caring the best you can for your employees. They are the heart and soul of everything we stand for. They offer caring and compassionate love to our friends who were unfortunate to be diagnosed with dementia. As a leader, your job is to be the wave of change by starting and continually improving and encouraging others, by example, by learning, teaching, coaching, and mentoring.

As I have mentioned before, the small breeze from the wings of a butterfly can implement change. That's why the cover of this book is an artist's rendering of a butterfly. It symbolizes that when we serve our friends diagnosed with dementia and implement small changes within ourselves, our leadership, and our team, those small changes will be reflected in how we serve our friends.

Are you prepared for the wave of dementia care that is coming? What small change are you implementing today? For yourself and your team?

With Peace and Blessings - Godspeed to You!

Christopher Smith
(C.A. Smith)

I am planning on workbooks, book summaries and more.
If you would like to be notified, sign up at
CASmithAuthor.com

If you enjoyed this book,
please leave a brief review on Amazon.
Best regards and thank you in advance:
Amazon.com/dp/B08RMRZVQY

Author Page
CASmithAuthor.com

Wellspring Senior Care

LinkedIn
LinkedIn.com/in/TheWellspringSenior

Facebook
Facebook.com/WellspringSeniorcare

Webpage
TheWellspringSenior.com/

WAG - Woodbridge Advisory Group

Facebook
Facebook.com/TheWAGpros

Webpage
WAGpros.com